Study Guide and Review Manual of
Human Embryology

5th EDITION

KEITH L. MOORE, PhD, FIAC, FRSM
Professor Emeritus of Anatomy and Cell Biology
Faculty of Medicine, University of Toronto
Toronto, Ontario, Canada

Professor of Human Anatomy and Cell Science
Department of Anatomy, Faculty of Medicine
University of Manitoba
Winnipeg, Manitoba, Canada

T.V.N. PERSAUD, MD, PhD, DSc, FRCPath (Lond.)
Professor and Former Head
Department of Human Anatomy and Cell Science
Professor of Pediatrics and Child Health
Professor of Obstetrics, Gynecology, and Reproductive Sciences
University of Manitoba, Faculty of Medicine

Consultant in Pathology and Clinical Genetics
Health Sciences Center
Winnipeg, Manitoba, Canada

W.B. SAUNDERS COMPANY
A Division of Harcourt Brace & Company
Philadelphia London Toronto Montreal Sydney Tokyo

W.B. SAUNDERS COMPANY
A Division of Harcourt Brace & Company

The Curtis Center
Independence Square West
Philadelphia, Pennsylvania 19106

Library of Congress Cataloging-in-Publication Data

Moore, Keith L.
Study guide and review manual of human embryology / Keith L. Moore,
T.V.N. Persaud.—5th ed.

p.   cm.

ISBN 0–7216–7378–3

1. Embryology, Human—Handbooks, manuals, etc.   I. Persaud,
   T. V. N.   II. Title.

QM601.M665   1998   612.6′4—dc21

97-33990

STUDY GUIDE AND REVIEW MANUAL OF HUMAN EMBRYOLOGY   ISBN 0-7216-7378-3

Copyright © 1998, 1993, 1988, 1982, 1975 by W.B. Saunders Company.

Printed in the United States of America.

Last digit is the print number: 9   8   7   6   5   4   3   2   1

Study Guide and Review Manual of

Human Embryology

*To our wives, children, and
grandchildren*

User's Guide

■ This study guide is designed to help you learn and later review human embryology by providing learning objectives and various types of multiple-choice questions based on these objectives. The guide is not intended as a substitute for careful study of your textbook and lecture notes; however, it is designed to enable you to detect areas of weakness and afford you the opportunity to correct deficits in your knowledge.

Although the answers to the questions are explained and relevant notes are given, you should consult your textbook for a comprehensive review of difficult concepts and processes. Through discussion of weak areas with your colleagues and instructors, you can test your ability to do the things listed as learning objectives. To use this guide most effectively, the following steps are suggested:

1. Read the objectives listed at the beginning of the chapter you plan to study.

2. Carefully study the appropriate chapter in your textbook, focusing on the topics included in the objectives.

3. Attempt the series of questions: five-choice completion and five-choice association. All questions are designed to be answered at the rate of about one per minute. As you complete each set of questions, check your answers. If any of your answers are wrong, read the notes and explanations and study the appropriate material and illustrations in your textbook before proceeding to the next set of questions.

4. If you get 80% or more of the questions correct on the first trial, or during a subsequent review, you have performed well and should have no difficulty answering similar questions based on the objectives given in this guide.

Preface

■ The fifth edition of the *Study Guide and Review Manual* is designed primarily for use with the authors' textbooks: *The Developing Human: Clinically Oriented Embryology* and *Before We Are Born: Essentials of Embryology and Birth Defects,* published by the W.B. Saunders Company; however, it can be used with similar advantage by students using other textbooks of human embryology. The questions deal with the essentials of human embryology and birth defects that are of practical value and are similar to those commonly used in national board examinations.

This book is designed as a *study guide for beginning students* and as a *review manual* for advanced students preparing for National Board of Medical Examiners USMLE and other examinations. Because multiple-choice examinations are used more and more, and are formidable even to the best prepared, commonly used types of these questions have been developed around each topic in embryology and teratology. The test questions are intended for those who wish to determine the state of their knowledge and to improve their skills with multiple-choice examinations. More clinically oriented questions and illustrations have been added to this edition.

With less time available for formal study of embryology, there is a need for more independent study by students. To learn independently, stated objectives are required. At the beginning of each chapter, there is a list of objectives indicating what students should be able to do when they have completed their study of the chapter. The self-assessment questions and answers in each chapter provide students with feedback as to their status in achieving the objectives and afford them the opportunity to correct deficits that may exist in their knowledge.

The letters and comments we have received from students around the world expressing their appreciation of this *Study Guide and Review Manual* stimulated us to update the manual. We are grateful to our students and colleagues for their help in improving the questions and answers. We welcome suggestions for new questions and improvement of old ones. We are especially grateful to Marion Moore, the senior author's wife, who typed the original manuscipt of the Study Guide and reviewed the manuscript for this edition.

KEITH L. MOORE
T.V.N. PERSAUD

Contents

Introduction to Human Embryology

Objectives
Be able to:

- Define the term development and name the developmental periods.*
- Differentiate between the terms conceptus and abortus.
- Explain why embryology forms a basis for medical and dental practice.
- Differentiate between the terms embryology and teratology.
- Use the various terms of position and direction, and illustrate the various planes of the body.
- Explain the difference in meaning between embryo and fetus, conception and conceptus, and embryology and developmental anatomy.

■ FIVE-CHOICE COMPLETION QUESTIONS

Directions: Each of the following statements or questions is followed by five suggested responses or completions. **Select the one best answer** in each case.

1. The term conceptus includes all structures that develop from the
   - A. chorion
   - B. embryoblast
   - C. zygote
   - D. trophoblast
   - E. inner cell mass

2. Select the best term for describing the foot with reference to the leg.
   - A. distal
   - B. ventral
   - C. posterior
   - D. inferior
   - E. proximal

3. A section through an embryo that divides it into ventral and dorsal parts is a _____ section.
   - A. cross
   - B. sagittal
   - C. frontal
   - D. oblique
   - E. median

---

*Make no attempt to memorize the Timetables of Human Prenatal Development. Use them as you would a calendar to indicate important events.

Five-Choice Completion Questions *Continued*

4. In the adult, the neck is superior to the thorax. The corresponding term for a fetus is
   - A. dorsal
   - B. inferior
   - C. caudal
   - D. ventral
   - E. cranial

5. The plane that divides a fetus into right and left halves is called the _____ plane.
   - A. sagittal
   - B. median
   - C. coronal
   - D. transverse
   - E. frontal

6. Which of the following embryological terms means toward the nose?
   - A. dorsal
   - B. cephalic
   - C. cranial
   - D. rostral
   - E. caudal

7. Each of the following terms of comparison is used correctly, *except:*
   - A. The wrist is distal to the forearm.
   - B. The brain is cranial to the spinal cord.
   - C. The upper limb arises caudal to the heart.
   - D. The knee is proximal to the ankle.
   - E. The tail of the embryo is caudal to the abdomen.

8. Primary induction is fundamental to all developmental processes. This was discovered by:
   - A. Wilhelm Roux
   - B. Leeuwenhoek
   - C. Hans Spemann
   - D. von Baer
   - E. Malpighi

9. From which of the following is the morula formed?
   - A. oocyte
   - B. sperm
   - C. zygote
   - D. blastocyst
   - E. gastrula

10. Each of the following statements concerning an abortion or pregnancy loss is correct *except:*
    - A. Pregnancy loss occurs during the embryonic period.
    - B. Pregnancy loss may occur after the eighth week of gestation
    - C. The aborted embryo or fetus is not viable.
    - D. The aborted conceptus is always expelled from the uterus.
    - E. Abortion may be clinically induced.

11. Embryonic development results from growth and differentiation of specialized cells. This was first suggested by
    - A. Hippocrates
    - B. William Harvey
    - C. Hans Spemann
    - D. Franklin P. Mall
    - E. Caspar Friedrich Wolff

■ ANSWERS AND EXPLANATIONS

1. **C**   The term conceptus is used when referring to the embryo (or fetus) and its membranes (i.e., the total products of conception that develop from the zygote). The conceptus (embryo and its membranes) that is expelled or removed during an abortion is called an abortus.

2. **A**   The foot is at the distal end of the leg. The term distal is commonly used in descriptions of a limb instead of the term inferior.

3. **C**   A vertical section through the coronal (frontal) plane is known as a coronal section. The coronal plane is a major plane of the body.

4. **E**   The neck of a fetus is cranial (cephalic) to the thorax; that is, it is closer to the head. Cranial means toward the cranium, and cephalic indicates toward the brain.

5. **B**   The median plane is a vertical plane that passes through the center of the body, dividing it into right and left halves. The median plane passes longitudinally through the embryo and intersects the surface of the front and back of the body at what are called the anterior and posterior median lines.

6. **D**   The term rostral is used to indicate the relation of structures to the nose (L. *rostrum,* a beak). For example, the philtrum of the lip develops rostral to the eye.

7. **C**   The upper limb arises opposite the heart. The Latin term *caudal* means toward the tail.

8. **C**   Hans Spemann (1869–1941) discovered the phenomenon of primary induction (i.e., how one tissue determines the fate of another). For this, he received the Nobel Prize in 1935. Over the decades, scientists have been attempting to isolate the substances that are transmitted from one tissue to another, causing induction. There is some evidence that endogenous retinoic acid is a likely morphogen that induces the normal pattern of embryonic structures.

9. **C**   Cleavage, or division, of the zygote gives rise to a ball of 12 to 16 blastomeres, called a morula. This occurs about 3 days after fertilization and precedes the formation of both the blastocyst and the gastrula.

10. **D**   Termination of pregnancy, whether naturally occurring or clinically induced, before 20 weeks of gestation is considered to be an abortion. The aborted embryo or fetus is not viable. In cases of missed abortion, after the embryo or fetus dies the product of conception is not expelled but retained in the uterus. Spontaneous abortions occur naturally during the first 12 weeks of pregnancy; many are not detected clinically, especially when they occur very early in pregnancy.

11. **E**   Caspar Friedrich Wolff proposed in his doctoral thesis, *Theoria generationis* (1759), that the embryo develops from layers of cells, derived from the division of the zygote. This concept led to the theory of epigenesis. Before this, it was believed that all structures of the embryo already exist in the sperm or fertilized oocyte, and during development it becomes a new organism by unfolding itself (preformation theory). William Harvey carried out comparative studies in embryology; Hans Spemann discovered the phenomenon of induction; and Franklin P. Mall collected and studied human embryos.

■ FIVE-CHOICE ASSOCIATION QUESTIONS

Directions: Each group of questions below consists of a numbered list of descriptive words or phrases accompanied by a diagram with certain parts indicated by letters or by a list of lettered headings. For each numbered word or phrase, **select the lettered part of the heading** that matches it correctly and then insert the letter in the space to the right of the appropriate number. Sometimes more than one numbered word or phrase may be correctly matched to the same lettered part or heading.

A. Median
B. Dorsal
C. Coronal

D. Caudal
E. Rostral

1. _____ Posterior
2. _____ Toward nose
3. _____ Frontal
4. _____ Midsagittal
5. _____ Toward tail
6. _____ Lying in middle

7. _____ Transverse plane
8. _____ Rostral
9. _____ Median plane
10. _____ Frontal plane
11. _____ Sagittal plane
12. _____ Coronal plane

■ ANSWERS AND EXPLANATIONS

1. **B** Dorsal refers to structures near the back. In the adult, dorsal is equivalent to posterior. The term dorsal is commonly used in descriptions of embryos and in some descriptions of embryos and in some descriptions of adults (e.g., we re-fer to the dorsum or the dorsal part of the foot and hand).

2. **E** Structures that are near the nose are rostral (e.g., a structure such as a nerve

Answers and Explanations *Continued*

grows rostrally (toward the nose) or in a rostral direction).

3. **C** The term coronal often is used synonymously with frontal. Coronal refers to the fact that a coronal plane passes through the coronal suture of the skull.

4. **A** A midsagittal section passes through the median plane. Thus, the terms midsagittal and median are used synonymously in reference to sections cut in the median plane, but the term median is preferable.

5. **D** Caudal is used in the description of structures that are near the tail or rump of the embryo. Embryos have tails until the early part of the eighth week. In descriptions of adult anatomy, the term inferior is used to indicate structures that are lower in the body (e.g., the large intestine is inferior to the stomach).

6. **A** Median means lying in the median plane or midline, and the term medial is used to indicate a structure nearer the median plane (e.g., the eye is medial to the auricle of the external ear).

7. **C** The transverse plane is any plane that is at right angles to both the median and the frontal plane. Although the term transverse often is used synonymously with horizontal, you must understand that transverse implies that it is through the longitudinal axis of a structure. In the anatomic position, a transverse section through the foot in the anatomic position

is coronal. Transverse sections commonly are used in embryology (e.g., serial transverse sections of chick and pig embryos often are studied in the laboratory).

8. **D** The term rostral (toward the nose) is used to indicate the relation of a structure to the nose (e.g., the eyes are rostral to the ears).

9. **B** The median plane is a vertical plane that passes through the center of the body, dividing it into right and left halves. Median sections of embryos show the relation of thoracic and abdominal structures to each other.

10. **E** A frontal plane is any vertical plane that intersects the median plane at a right angle. This kind of section is helpful in studying paired structures (e.g., the kidneys) and those that run longitudinally (e.g., the esophagus).

11. **A** A sagittal plane is any vertical plane that passes through the body parallel to the median plane. A median section passes through the median plane. These sections often are used to show the course of structures that run through various regions of the body (e.g., the esophagus runs through the neck and thorax).

12. **E** A frontal plane often is called a coronal plane because a frontal plane passes through the coronal suture of the skull. It divides the body into ventral and dorsal parts. Sections through the frontal plane commonly are used in studying embryos.

■ NOTES

Beginnings of Human Development

2

Objectives

Be able to:

- Describe spermatogenesis and oogenesis with special emphasis on the chromosomal changes that occur during maturation of the germ cells.
- Compare the sperm and the oocyte (ovum) with reference to size, chromosome constitution, time of formation, transport, and viability.
- Define the term nondisjunction, and explain how this abnormal process leads to monosomy and trisomy. Describe the most common syndrome that results from nondisjunction.
- Discuss the ovarian cycle (follicle development, ovulation, and corpus luteum formation) and the menstrual cycle, explaining how ovarian cyclic activity is intimately linked with cyclic changes in the endometrium.
- Discuss capacitation and the acrosome reaction of the sperm.
- Construct and label simple diagrams showing fertilization. List the results of fertilization.
- Discuss cleavage of the zygote and implantation of the blastocyst, using labeled sketches. Define blastocyst, zona pellucida, trophoblast, inner cell mass, blastocyst cavity, embryonic pole, embryoblast, blastocyst cavity, and hypoblast.

■ FIVE-CHOICE COMPLETION QUESTIONS

Directions: Each of the following statements or questions is followed by five suggested responses or completions. **Select the one best answer** in each case.

1. Before ejaculation, sperm are stored chiefly in the
   - A. seminal vesicles
   - B. efferent ductules
   - C. ejaculatory ducts
   - D. epididymis
   - E. rete testis

2. Which of the following types of germ cell does not undergo cell division?
   - A. spermatogonia
   - B. primary oocytes
   - C. spermatids
   - D. secondary spermatocytes
   - E. oogonia

Five-Choice Completion Questions *Continued*

3. Which of the following chromosomal constitutions in a sperm normally results in a male, if it fertilizes an ovum?

   A. 22, O
   B. 22, X
   C. 22, Y

   D. 23, X
   E. 23, Y

4. Oogonia are homologous to spermatogonia. They divide by mitosis during

   A. all postnatal periods
   B. early fetal life
   C. puberty

   D. the reproductive period
   E. none of the above

5. The normal chromosome number of a human spermatid is

   A. 23 autosomes plus 2 different sex chromosomes
   B. 22 autosomes plus an X and a Y chromosome
   C. 23 autosomes plus 2 identical sex chromosomes
   D. 22 autosomes plus an X or a Y chromosome
   E. 46, XY

6. Morphologically abnormal sperm may cause

   A. monosomy
   B. congenital anomalies
   C. trisomy

   D. abnormal embryos
   E. infertility

7. Which of the following layers of the embryo is recognizable at the end of the first week of development?

   A. hypoblast
   B. mesoderm
   C. ectoderm

   D. epiblast
   E. somatopleure

8. The secondary oocyte completes the second meiotic division

   A. before ovulation
   B. during ovulation
   C. at fertilization

   D. before birth
   E. at puberty

9. The sperm penetrates the zona pellucida, digesting a path by the action of enzymes released from the _____ of the sperm.

   A. middle piece
   B. acrosome
   C. neck

   D. main piece
   E. head

10. How many sperm would probably be deposited by a normal young adult male in the vagina during intercourse?

    A. 300 thousand
    B. 3 million
    C. 30 million

    D. 300 million
    E. 3 billion

Five-Choice Completion Questions *Continued*

11. A 42-year-old woman became pregnant. She was concerned about the health of her unborn child and consulted a physician. There is a risk for which of the following?

    A. intrauterine growth retardation
    B. gene mutation
    C. chromosomal abnormalities
    D. miscarriage
    E. premature birth

12. Freshly ejaculated sperm are not capable of fertilizing oocytes because these sperm are:

    A. inactive
    B. not yet capacitated
    C. morphologically abnormal
    D. immature
    E. very motile

13. Routine ultrasound examination of a pregnant woman revealed the presence of 12 live embryos. (This is a true clinical case.) Which of the following is the probable cause?

    A. The inner cell mass has divided into 12 independent embryos.
    B. Progesterone secretion is increased.
    C. The woman was treated with an antifertility drug.
    D. Twelve oocytes were fertilized by 12 sperm.
    E. Release of gonadotropins is inadequate.

14. The semen of a man believed to be responsible for a sterile marriage was evaluated. Which of the following is of least importance in assessing the man's fertility?

    A. sperm count
    B. morphology of the sperm
    C. zinc concentration of semen
    D. calcium ions
    E. sperm motility

15. During spermatogenesis, which of the following undergoes a second meiotic division?

    A. spermatogonia
    B. primary spermatocytes
    C. secondary spermatocytes
    D. spermatids
    E. spermatozoa

16. An infant is diagnosed as having 47 chromosomes instead of 46. This abnormal condition (trisomy) results from

    A. gene mutation
    B. nondisjunction
    C. disturbances in spermiogenesis
    D. disturbances in mitosis
    E. abnormal spermatogonia

■ ANSWERS AND EXPLANATIONS

1. **D**   Sperm are stored and undergo further maturation in the epididymis. They are not stored in the seminal vesicles, as was believed for many years. During ejaculation, the sperm are forced through the ductus deferens into the urethra, from which they are expelled with the secretions of the accessory glands (e.g., the prostate) as semen. If not ejaculated, the sperm degenerate and are absorbed within the epididymis.

2. **C**   Spermatids do not divide. They are gradually transformed into mature sperm during spermiogenesis.

3. **E**   Fertilization of an ovum by a Y sperm (i.e., 23,Y) produces a 46,XY zygote that normally develops into a male. The number 46 designates the total number of chromosomes, including the two sex chromosomes (XY). This is the accepted way of indicating the chromosomal composition of cells. The sex of the embryo depends on whether an X or a Y sperm fertilizes the ovum. The mother can contribute only an X chromosome and so cannot determine the embryo's sex.

4. **B**   Oogonia proliferate during the early fetal period and, unlike spermatogonia, do not begin to increase at puberty. All oogonia become primary oocytes before birth. Many of the 2 million or so oocytes present in both ovaries at birth degenerate before puberty, leaving not more than 40,000 to undergo further development after puberty.

5. **D**   Spermatids are haploid cells (23 chromosomes) that have 22 autosomes plus a Y or an X chromosome (i.e., one or the other but not both). Thus, the haploid number in humans is 23. If two members of a chromosome pair fail to separate (nondisjunction), abnormal spermatids can have 22 autosomes and 2 sex chromosomes, or no sex chromosome.

6. **E**   It is believed that structurally abnormal sperm do not fertilize ova because of their lack of normal motility and fertilizing power. Examination of semen is important in the study of fertility. The number, motility, and abnormalities in size and shape of sperm are important in assessing sterility in males. If 20% or more sperm are morphologically abnormal, fertility usually is impaired.

7. **A**   The bilaminar embryonic disc forms early in the second week. At the end of the first week, the hypoblast (primordial endoderm) begins to form on the ventral surface of the inner cell mass. It has been suggested that the hypoblast is derived from the inner cell mass by delamination. The epiblast, which gives rise to the embryonic ectoderm and mesoderm, is not recognizable until the beginning of the second week, when the amniotic cavity forms.

8. **C**   When a sperm contacts the cell membrane of a secondary oocyte, the oocyte completes the second maturation or meiotic division and becomes a mature ovum or oocyte. The second polar body, a nonfunctional cell, is formed during this division. If fertilization does not occur, the secondary oocyte does not complete this division; it degenerates within 24 hours after ovulation.

9. **B**   It is believed that the sperm digests a path for itself through the corona radiata by the action of enzymes, including hyaluronidase, released from the sperm's acrosome through perforations that develop in it during the acrosome reaction. Tubal mucosal enzymes appear to assist hyaluronidase. Acrosomal enzymes, especially acrosin, are also important for the penetration of the zona pellucida. Movements of the tail of the sperm may be involved in this process.

10. **D**   At least 300 million sperm are deposited in the vagina during sexual intercourse. Usually 200 million to 600 million sperm are in the ejaculate, but only

Answers and Explanations *Continued*

a few hundred sperm are believed to reach the fertilization site. If less than 50 million sperm are present in a semen sample, the male from whom the sample was taken may be infertile.

11. **C** The incidence of children with trisomy 21 or Down syndrome increases with maternal age. Because of the woman's advanced age, the primary oocytes have been dormant in arrested first meiotic division for about 30 years. During meiosis, sometimes homologous chromosomes fail to separate and migrate to opposite poles of the cell, a condition known as nondisjunction. The result is that some germ cells have 24 chromosomes instead of 23, and others have only 22. Trisomy occurs when a gamete with 24 chromosomes fuses with a normal one during fertilization, forming a zygote with 47 chromosomes. Children born with Down syndrome have a characteristic facial appearance and are mentally retarded.

12. **B** Glycoproteins and seminal proteins on the surface of the acrosome of freshly ejaculated sperm must first be removed to facilitate fertilization of the oocyte. This process, which lasts about 7 hours, is known as capacitation and usually occurs in the uterus or uterine tubes. Capacitated sperm are more active.

13. **D** The woman probably was treated with fertility drugs (e.g., gonadotropins, clomiphene citrate) to stimulate ovulation. The incidence of multiple pregnancy increases considerably when ovulation is stimulated with gonadotropins or an ovulatory agent. The relatively large number of embryos present probably resulted from the fertilization of that many mature oocytes by individual sperm.

14. **C** Zinc concentrations of the male reproductive organs are relatively high, but there is no difference in zinc concentrations of seminal fluid from fertile and infertile men. In normal males, there are more than 100 million sperm per milliliter of semen. Less than 10 million sperm per milliliter of semen are likely to be from someone who is sterile, especially if there are immotile and abnormal sperm in the specimen. As many as 18 per cent of the sperm in an ejaculate may be abnormal without affecting fertility. Calcium ions in the semen, like prostaglandins, are involved in the movement of sperm.

15. **C** Secondary spermatocytes undergo a second meiotic division to form spermatids, which subsequently are transformed into mature spermatozoa. Spermatogonia grow and give rise to the primary spermatocytes by mitotic division. Each primary spermatocyte then undergoes the first meiotic division to form two secondary spermatocytes with a haploid chromosomal complement.

16. **B** Trisomy is a relatively common numerical chromosomal anomaly resulting from an error in meiotic cell division during gametogenesis. When homologous chromosomes fail to separate and migrate to opposite poles of the germ cell, some gametes have 24 chromosomes and others have 22. This abnormal condition is known as *nondisjunction*. In the event of fertilization occurring between a gamete with 24 chromosomes and a normal gamete with 23 chromosomes, the resulting zygote has 47 chromosomes (trisomy). Spermatogonia are the primitive male germ cells with a chromosomal constitution of 46, XY, and they give rise to the spermatozoa. Spermatids differentiate into mature spermatozoa by a process known as spermiogenesis.

■ FIVE-CHOICE ASSOCIATION QUESTIONS

Directions: Each group of questions below consists of a numbered list of descriptive words or phrases accompanied by a diagram with certain parts indicated by letters or by a list of lettered headings. For each numbered word or phrase, **select the lettered part or heading** that matches it correctly and then insert the letter in the space to the right of the appropriate number. Sometimes more than one numbered word or phrase may be correctly matched to the same lettered part or heading.

A. Polar bodies
B. Capacitation
C. Acrosome

D. Zona pellucida
E. Pronuclei

1. _____ Haploid nuclei that fuse to form a zygote
2. _____ Changes occur in it that inhibit entry of sperm
3. _____ Contains enzymes that digest a path for the sperm
4. _____ Nonfunctional cells produced during oogenesis

5. _____ Polar body
6. _____ Zona pellucida
7. _____ Diploid cells
8. _____ Meiotic spindle
9. _____ Corona radiata
10. _____ Haploid cell

11. _____ Embryoblast
12. _____ Gives rise to part of the placenta
13. _____ Gives rise to the embryo
14. _____ Gives rise to the hypoblast
15. _____ Degenerates and disappears
16. _____ Blastocyst cavity

Five-Choice Association Questions *Continued*

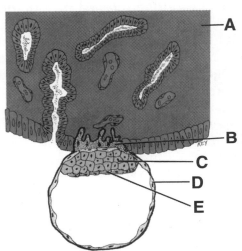

17. _____ Once filled the follicular antrum
18. _____ Develops under luteinizing hormone influence
19. _____ Produces progesterone
20. _____ Expelled with the follicular fluid
21. _____ Fimbriae
22. _____ Derived from a primary oocyte

23. _____ Cytotrophoblast
24. _____ Inner cell mass
25. _____ Endometrium
26. _____ Hypoblast
27. _____ Syncytiotrophoblast

■ ANSWERS AND EXPLANATIONS

1. **E** The male and female pronuclei are the haploid nuclei of the sperm and the ovum, respectively. They fuse during fertilization to form the diploid nucleus of a zygote. The nucleus occupies most of the head of the sperm, and after it enters the ovum, it swells to form the male pronucleus. The pronuclei are about equal in size and show similar features.

2. **D** The zona pellucida undergoes changes, called the zona reaction, when a sperm contacts the cell membrane of a secondary oocyte. These changes, caused by the release of substances from the oo-

cyte, prevent other sperm from passing through the zona pellucida and entering the oocyte.

3. **C** The acrosome is a caplike structure that invests the anterior half of the head of the sperm. It contains enzymes that pass through perforations in its wall and digest a path for the sperm to follow through the zona pellucida to contact the oocyte.

4. **A** The polar bodies are small haploid cells produced during the first and second meiotic divisions. The polar bodies

Answers and Explanations *Continued*

have the same number of chromosomes as the secondary and mature oocytes, but they receive little cytoplasm. Most cytoplasm goes to the mature oocyte, which, if fertilized, contributes to the zygote. The sperm probably does not contribute any cytoplasm to the zygote.

5. **D** The first polar body forms during the first meiotic division. Note that it is inside the zona pellucida with the secondary oocyte. The polar body is a haploid cell and receives little cytoplasm. Although it may divide into two polar bodies, all these cells degenerate. The secondary oocyte receives the same number of chromosomes as the polar body; however, it gets almost all the cytoplasm.

6. **C** The zona pellucida surrounds the secondary oocyte and the polar body. This membrane is surrounded by a layer of follicular cells called the corona radiata. The zona pellucida appears homogeneous in the fresh condition, but under the electron microscope it appears granular and shows some concentric layering.

7. **A** The follicular cells of the corona radiata are the only diploid cells in the diagram. During follicular development, the follicular cells proliferate by mitosis and form a stratified epithelium around the oocyte. In the mature follicle, the oocyte lies in a mound of follicular cells, called the cumulus oophorus. When the oocyte is expelled at ovulation, it is surrounded by the zona pellucida and one or more layers of follicular cells, as shown in the diagram.

8. **E** Contact of a sperm with the cell membrane of the oocyte stimulates the secondary oocyte to complete its second meiotic division. This contact also brings about the zona reaction, preventing entry of more sperm. The sperm penetrates the cell membrane of the secondary oocyte and then passes into the cyto-

plasm of the oocyte, leaving its cell membrane outside the oocyte.

9. **A** As previously described, the corona radiata consists of one or more layers of follicular cells that surround the zona pellucida, the polar body, and the secondary oocyte. The corona radiata is dispersed during fertilization by enzymes released from the acrosomes of the sperm that surround the ovum.

10. **D** The first polar body is a haploid cell formed during the first meiotic division of the oocyte. The sperm is also a haploid cell. The sex chromosomal content of the sperm determines the sex of the zygote. If a sperm with an X chromosome fertilizes an ovum, a zygote forms that normally develops into a female. If a sperm with a Y chromosome fertilizes an ovum, a zygote forms that normally develops into a male. Because there are equal numbers of X and Y sperm, the chances of a male or female zygote resulting from fertilization are equal. Despite this, more males than females are born.

11. **B** The embryoblast or inner cell mass is recognizable about 4 days after fertilization. It is derived from the central cells of the morula. The embryoblast gives rise to the embryo.

12. **D** The outer cell layer of the blastocyst (trophoblast) gives rise to the embryonic part of the placenta; the other part is derived from the endometrium. When the trophoblast becomes lined by extraembryonic somatic mesoderm, the combined layers are called the chorion. The trophoblast forms no part of the embryo.

13. **B** The embryoblast, or inner cell mass, gives rise to the embryo. The first sign of differentiation of the inner cell mass is the appearance of the hypoblast on its ventral surface. The inner cell mass later gives rise to two more germ layers. The

Answers and Explanations *Continued*

three germ layers give rise to all the tissues and organs of the embryo.

14. **B** At the end of the first week, differentiation of the inner cell mass gives rise to the hypoblast. It appears as a flattened layer on the ventral surface of the inner cell mass. Later, it forms the roof of the yolk sac and is incorporated into the embryo as the lining of the primitive gut.

15. **A** The zona pellucida begins to degenerate about 4 days after fertilization as the blastocyst begins to expand rapidly. The zona pellucida disappears on the fourth or fifth day. Implantation begins on the sixth day.

16. **C** The blastocyst cavity forms as fluid passes into the morula from the uterus and accumulates. The spaces around the central cells of the morula coalesce to form the blastocyst cavity, converting the morula into a blastocyst. The uterine fluid in the blastocyst cavity bathes the ventral surface of the inner cell mass and probably supplies nutrients to the embryonic cells.

17. **C** Follicular fluid fills the antra of growing and mature ovarian follicles. When the stigma ruptures at ovulation, the oocyte is expelled with the fluid from the follicle and the ovary in a few seconds. The expulsion of the ovum and the fluid is the result of intrafollicular pressure and, possibly, ovarian smooth muscle contraction.

18. **E** The corpus luteum develops under the influence of the luteinizing hormone. It produces progesterone and some estrogen. These hormones act on the endometrium, bringing about the secretory phase and preparing the endometrium for implantation of a blastocyst. If the ovum is fertilized, the corpus luteum enlarges into a corpus luteum of pregnancy and increases its hormone production. If the ovum is not fertilized, the corpus luteum

begins to degenerate about 9 days after ovulation and is called a corpus luteum of menstruation.

19. **E** The corpus luteum usually produces progesterone for about 9 days. If the ovum is fertilized, it produces progesterone until about the end of the fourth month of pregnancy. If you chose **A** for the answer, you are partly right because the ovary produces progesterone. **E** is a better answer because it is more specific.

20. **B** The secondary oocyte is expelled with follicular fluid at ovulation. Ovulation is under follicle-stimulating hormone and luteinizing hormone influence and occurs through the ruptured stigma. The oocyte quickly leaves the peritoneal cavity and enters the infundibulum (L. funnel) of the uterine tube.

21. **D** The fimbriae of the uterine tube embrace the ovary at ovulation. The sweeping motion of the fimbriae and the motion of the cilia on their epithelial lining cells carry the oocyte into the uterine tube.

22. **B** The secondary oocyte is derived from a primary oocyte after the first meiotic division. This division produces two haploid cells, the secondary oocyte and the first polar body. By the time of ovulation, the secondary oocyte has begun the second meiotic division but progresses only to the metaphase stage, where division is arrested. If the oocyte is fertilized, it completes the division, forming a mature ovum.

23. **D** The trophoblast of the implanting blastocyst differentiates into two layers. The internal layer is known as the cytotrophoblast. Rapid proliferation of cells of the cytotrophoblast give rise to the syncytiotrophoblast, an outer layer of multinucleated cytoplasmic mass.

24. **C** The inner cell mass or embryoblast gives rise to the embryo. It arises from

Answers and Explanations *Continued*

cells that have segregated from the morula. This occurs about 4 days after fertilization. The remaining cells of the morula become the trophoblast of the blastocyst.

25. **A**   The blastocyst attaches to the epithelium covering the compact layer of the endometrium about 6 days after fertilization. The endometrium is in the secretory phase of the uterine cycle, with abundant blood vessels and secreting glands. The endometrial cells are enlarged and filled with glycogen as well as lipids.

26. **E**   The hypoblast appears at about 7 days after fertilization. It is a flattened layer of cells on the surface of the inner cell mass facing the blastocyst cavity. The hypoblast gives rise to the embryonic endoderm and the endoderm of the yolk sac.

27. **B**   The syncytiotrophoblast, like the cytotrophoblast, is derived from the trophoblast. The trophoblast proliferates rapidly following implantation, giving rise to these two layers. The syncytiotrophoblast is a multinucleated cytoplasmic mass with no discernible cell boundaries. The syncytiotrophoblast invades the uterine endometrium and facilitates the implantation of the blastocyst.

■ NOTES

Formation of the Bilaminar Embryonic Disc and Chorionic Sac

3

Objectives

Be able to:

- Describe implantation of a blastocyst, using simple, labeled diagrams.
- Discuss proliferation and differentiation of the trophoblast, formation of lacunar networks, and the establishment of the primitive uteroplacental circulation.
- Trace the development of the amniotic cavity, the bilaminar embryonic disc, the yolk sac, the extraembryonic mesoderm, the extraembryonic coelom, and the connecting stalk.
- Write brief notes on the prechordal plate, embryotroph, chorion, primary chorionic villi, chorionic sac, decidual reaction, and ectopic pregnancies.

■ FIVE-CHOICE COMPLETION QUESTIONS

Directions: Each of the following statements or questions is followed by five suggested responses or completions. **Select the one best answer** in each case.

1. The 8-day blastocyst
   A. has a single layer of trophoblast at the embryonic pole
   B. has lacunae in the syncytiotrophoblast
   C. is partially implanted in the endometrium
   D. is covered by the uterine epithelium
   E. has a primordial yolk sac

2. The syncytiotrophoblast
   A. surrounds the 8-day blastocyst
   B. has well-defined cell boundaries
   C. shows little invasive activity
   D. is derived from the cytotrophoblast
   E. is nonfunctional

Five-Choice Completion Questions *Continued*

3. The amniotic cavity develops

   A. initially on the 10th day
   B. within the exocoelomic cavity
   C. between the embryonic disc and the trophoblast
   D. in the extraembryonic mesoderm
   E. during the first week

4. Which statement about the 14-day blastocyst is *false*?

   A. Primary chorionic villi are absent.
   B. Extraembryonic coelom surrounds the yolk sac.
   C. The primordial uteroplacental circulation is established.
   D. The extraembryonic mesoderm is split into two layers.
   E. It is completely implanted in the endometrium.

5. In the 10- to 12-day blastocyst,

   A. the conceptus lies deep to the endometrial epithelium
   B. the defect in the endometrial epithelium is indicated by a closing plug
   C. the implanted blastocyst produces an elevation on the endometrial surface
   D. maternal blood begins to flow slowly through the lacunar networks
   E. all the above are correct

6. The wall of the chorionic sac is composed of

   A. cytotrophoblast and syncytiotrophoblast
   B. two layers of trophoblast lined by extraembryonic somatic mesoderm
   C. trophoblast and the exocoelomic membrane
   D. extraembryonic splanchnic mesoderm and both layers of trophoblast
   E. none of the above is correct

7. During the second week, lacunar networks develop within the

   A. extraembryonic mesoderm
   B. inner cell mass
   C. syncytiotrophoblast
   D. endometrium
   E. embryoblast

8. Ectopic implantations most commonly occur in the

   A. ovary
   B. abdomen
   C. uterine tube
   D. cervix
   E. peritoneal cavity

Five-Choice Completion Questions *Continued*

9. Each of the following is directly involved with early implantation, *except:*
   A. decidual reaction
   B. progesterone
   C. stratum spongiosum
   D. invasion
   E. endometrial epithelium

10. The amniotic cavity appears on the eighth day as a slitlike space between the trophoblast and the
   A. extraembryonic mesoderm
   B. inner cell mass
   C. exocoelomic membrane
   D. connecting stalk
   E. chorion

11. A 32-year-old woman was admitted to hospital because of abdominal pain and hemorrhage. Her last menstrual period was about 7 weeks earlier. Which of the following is the most likely diagnosis?
   A. appendicitis
   B. ovarian cyst
   C. miscarriage
   D. ectopic pregnancy
   E. placenta previa

12. During the second week of development, all the following structures are formed, *except* for the
   A. amniotic cavity
   B. neural plate
   C. yolk sac
   D. connecting stalk
   E. chorion

■ ANSWERS AND EXPLANATIONS

1. **C** The 8-day blastocyst is partially implanted in the endometrium. The trophoblast at the pole opposite the embryo (abembryonic pole) remains relatively undifferentiated, consisting of a thin layer of flattened cytotrophoblastic cells. The trophoblast consists of two layers only where it is in contact with the endometrium (usually adjacent to the inner cell mass). The primitive yolk sac is not usually present at 8 days, but the amniotic cavity is represented by a small, slitlike space.

2. **D** The syncytiotrophoblast is derived from the cytotrophoblast. The cytotrophoblast is mitotically active and forms new cells that fuse with and become part of the increasing mass of syncytiotrophoblast. The syncytiotrophoblast does not enclose the 8-day blastocyst on all sides.

It forms a multinucleated cytoplasmic mass at the embryonic pole. The syncytiotrophoblast does not have well-defined cell boundaries. Invasiveness is one of the spectacular properties of the syncytiotrophoblast. The penetration and subsequent erosion of the endometrium by the syncytiotrophoblast results from proteolytic enzymes produced by the syncytiotrophoblast.

3. **C** The amniotic cavity appears as a small cavity in the inner cell mass on the eighth day after fertilization between the embryonic disc and the invading syncytiotrophoblast. It does not develop in the exocoelomic cavity or in the extraembryonic mesoderm. The amnion forms from cells derived from the epiblast.

4. **A** Primary chorionic villi are characteristic features of the 14-day blastocyst. All

Answers and Explanations *Continued*

the other statements about the blastocyst at the end of the second week are true.

5. **E**   These statements about the 10- to 12-day blastocyst are all true. The important statement is **D** because the presence of maternal blood establishes an abundant source of nutrition for the conceptus.

6. **B**   The wall of the chorionic sac is composed of the chorion, which is formed by the combination of extraembryonic somatic mesoderm and the two layers of trophoblast (cytotrophoblast and syncytiotrophoblast). The chorionic sac contains the embryo, which is attached to its wall by the connecting stalk.

7. **C**   Lacunar networks develop in the syncytiotrophoblast by coalescence of lacunae (spaces). They do not form in the endometrium or in the inner cell mass. Although spaces or cavities form in the extraembryonic mesoderm, they are not called lacunae and they do not form lacunar networks. These extraembryonic coelomic spaces become confluent to form the extraembryonic coelom.

8. **C**   Ectopic, or extrauterine, pregnancies usually occur in the ampulla of the uterine tube. They are related to factors that delay or prevent passage of the morula to the uterus. Tubal rupture may be followed by early expulsion of a tubal pregnancy and secondary implantation of the blastocyst in the ovary or abdomen. Ectopic pregnancies, other than those in the tube, are rare. Cervical implantations are not ectopic (outside the uterus), but they are abnormal. Cervical implantations, usually in the superior part of the cervix, are uncommon. Cervical pregnancy is a serious complication of pregnancy because the placenta firmly attaches to the smooth muscle fibers of the cervix.

9. **C**   The stratum spongiosum of the endometrium is not directly involved with

early implantation. It does become involved with formation of the placenta later in pregnancy. The decidual reaction is the series of changes that occur in the endometrium as a result of implantation. It is believed that the blastocyst produces hormone-like substances that cause the decidual changes. Progesterone produced by the corpus luteum is the hormone believed to control implantation. Invasion of the endometrium by the syncytiotrophoblast is the most striking event that occurs during implantation. The trophoblast produces proteolytic enzymes that erode the epithelial cells of the endometrium and its connective tissues, glands, and blood vessels.

10. **B**   The amniotic cavity appears as a space between the trophoblast and the epiblast of the bilaminar embryonic disc. Attachment of the blastocyst to the endometrium usually occurs at the embryonic pole; hence, this area sometimes is called the polar trophoblast. The amniotic cavity does not develop between the extraembryonic mesoderm (or the connecting stalk) and the trophoblast.

11. **D**   The clinical symptoms, as well as the missed menstrual period, suggest an ectopic pregnancy (i.e., the blastocyst is implanted outside the uterine cavity). More than 90% of ectopic implantations occur in the uterine tubes, the majority in the ampulla or infundibulum. Rupture of the uterine tube and hemorrhage are serious complications. To prevent this, the affected tube and conceptus are surgically removed.

12. **B**   The neural plate is induced during the third week of development from epiblast cells. The epiblast and hypoblast of the bilaminar embryonic disc are derived from the inner cell mass during the second week of development. The amniotic cavity, yolk cavity, connecting stalk, and chorion are also formed during this period of development.

■ FIVE-CHOICE ASSOCIATION QUESTIONS

Directions: Each group of questions below consists of a numbered list of descriptive words or phrases accompanied by a diagram with certain parts indicated by letters or by a list of lettered headings. For each numbered word or phrase, **select the lettered part or heading** that matches it correctly and then insert the letter in the space to the right of the appropriate number. Sometimes more than one numbered word or phrase may be correctly matched to the same lettered part or heading.

1. _____ Extraembryonic coelom
2. _____ Contains embryotroph
3. _____ Cytotrophoblast
4. _____ Lacunar network
5. _____ Epiblast forms its floor
6. _____ Frequently occurs in the uterine tube
7. _____ Develops as a localized thickening of the hypoblast
8. _____ Develops from a ruptured ovarian follicle
9. _____ Surrounds the embryo and its amnion and yolk sac
10. _____ Enlarges as soon as implantation of a blastocyst occurs

A. Corpus luteum
B. Zona pellucida
C. Prechordal plate

D. Ectopic implantation
E. Chorionic sac

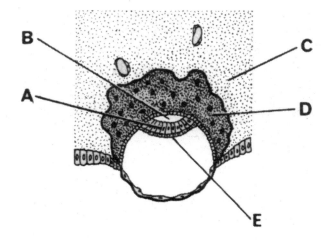

11. _____ Derived from cytotrophoblast
12. _____ Ventral layer of embryonic disc
13. _____ Site of the decidual reaction
14. _____ Multinucleated mass of cytoplasm
15. _____ Lies between the cytotrophoblast and the epiblast

Five-Choice Association Questions *Continued*

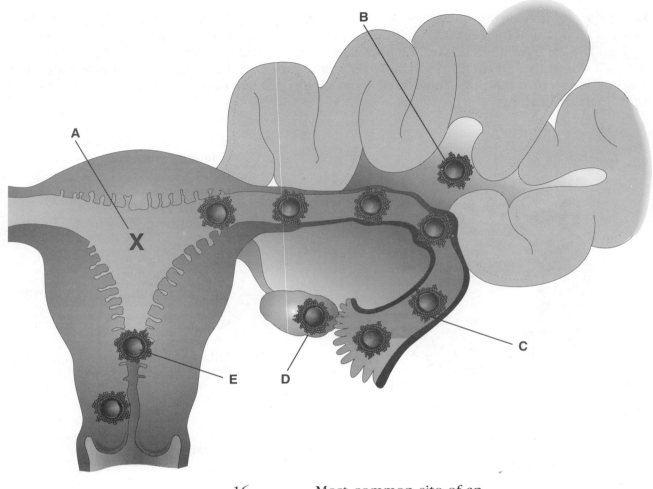

16. _____ Most common site of an ectopic pregnancy
17. _____ Abdominal pregnancy
18. _____ Usual site of implantation
19. _____ Implantation at internal os
20. _____ Ovarian pregnancy

■ ANSWERS AND EXPLANATIONS

1. **E** The extraembryonic coelom, part of which is indicated in the diagram, consists of isolated spaces in the extraembryonic mesoderm. Later, these spaces fuse or coalesce to form a single, large cavity known as the extraembryonic coelom.

2. **A** The lacunar networks (future intervillous space) contain a nutrient material

known as embryotroph. It is required by the embryo for growth and differentiation. Embryotroph consists of maternal blood, degenerated decidual cells, blood vessels, and glandular tissue.

3. **D** The cytotrophoblast is the inner layer of the trophoblast. It gives rise to (1) the outer layer of trophoblast (syncytiotro-

Answers and Explanations *Continued*

phoblast), (2) amnioblasts (cells that form the amnion), and (3) the extraembryonic mesoderm. The cytotrophoblast, as the prefix *cyto* implies, is a cellular layer.

4. **A** The lacunar networks form by coalescence of spaces in the syncytiotrophoblast. As the maternal sinusoids are eroded, blood seeps into these networks. Nutrients in the embryotroph diffuse through the two layers of trophoblast and pass to the embryo by way of the extraembryonic coelom.

5. **B** The floor of the amniotic cavity consists of embryonic epiblast. The amnion enclosing the amniotic cavity is attached to the epiblast of the embryonic disc. Initially, some amniotic fluid may be secreted by the amniotic cells, but most of it is derived from the maternal blood.

6. **D** Ectopic implantations usually occur in the uterine tube, most frequently in the ampulla, where fertilization normally occurs. Other sites of ectopic (outside the uterus) implantations are in the ovary and on the abdominal peritoneum.

7. **C** The prechordal plate indicates the future cranial end of the embryo and the future site of the mouth. It is a circular area that is firmly adherent to the overlying embryonic epiblast. It is an important landmark in the early embryo and seems to serve as an organizer of the cranial region of the embryo.

8. **A** The corpus luteum develops from the ovarian follicle after ovulation. Under the influence of luteinizing hormone produced by the hypophysis (anterior pituitary gland), the ruptured follicle develops into a glandular structure. At ovulation, the walls of the follicle collapse and, with cells of the theca folliculi, form the corpus luteum. The corpus luteum is an important source of progesterone for about 4 months. After this, the

placenta is the major producer of this hormone.

9. **E** The chorion forms a chorionic sac from the wall of which the embryo, its amnion, and yolk sac are suspended by the connecting stalk. The chorion gives rise to the embryonic part of the placenta. The maternal part of the placenta develops from the endometrium (decidua basalis).

10. **A** If an ovum is fertilized and the blastocyst implants, the corpus luteum enlarges to form a corpus luteum of pregnancy and increases its production of progesterone. This hormone is necessary for the maintenance of pregnancy. The corpus luteum is an important source of progesterone during the first trimester (3 months); it also produces estrogen. In later pregnancy, these hormones are produced by the placenta.

11. **D** The syncytiotrophoblast is derived from the cytotrophoblast. Cells of the cytotrophoblast divide mitotically, and some of these cells move outward, where they fuse with and become part of the increasing mass of syncytiotrophoblast. The syncytiotrophoblast produces human chorionic gonadotropin, which acts like luteinizing hormone in maintaining the corpus luteum. Later, it also produces other hormones.

12. **E** The hypoblast (primordial endoderm) forms the ventral layer of the embryonic disc. It is the primitive endoderm of the embryo. It is first recognizable on the ventral surface of the inner cell mass about 7 days after fertilization.

13. **C** The stroma (connective tissue) in the compact layer of the endometrium in the region of the implanting blastocyst is the site of cellular and other changes known as the decidual reaction. The enlarged cells, called decidual cells, contain large

Answers and Explanations *Continued*

amounts of glycogen and lipids that provide nourishment for the embryo.

14. **D**   The syncytiotrophoblast is a multinucleated protoplasmic mass derived by division of cytotrophoblast cells. This layer is devoid of cell boundaries. The syncytiotrophoblast is actively involved during implantation and produces substances that cause the decidual reaction. Later, this layer produces two protein hormones and two steroid hormones.

15. **B**   The amniotic cavity lies between the cytotrophoblast at the embryonic pole and the embryonic epiblast of the embryonic disc. Cells from the epiblast (amnioblasts) soon form a thin roof over this cavity called the amnion. It is continuous with the epiblast of the embryonic disc.

16. **C**   A pregnancy in which the blastocyst implants outside the uterine cavity is known as an ectopic pregnancy. The most common site of an ectopic pregnancy is the uterine tube, usually in the ampulla or isthmus. The incidence of tubal pregnancy ranges from 1 in 80 to 1 in 250 pregnancies, depending on the geographic location, socioeconomic level, and age of the pregnant woman. Pelvic inflammatory disease is a common cause of tubal ectopic pregnancy. If the tubal pregnancy is present on the right side, it should not be misdiagnosed as appendicitis. As the embryo increases in size, the uterine tube ruptures, leading to hemorrhage and a serious threat to the mother's life.

17. **B**   In an abdominal pregnancy, the conceptus develops on the peritoneal surfaces of the abdominal cavity. Abdominal pregnancies are relatively uncommon (about 0.03% of all ectopic pregnancies), and they are usually associated with intra-abdominal hemorrhage and severe abdominal pain. Rarely the embryo continues to develop until term and a live fetus may be delivered surgically. In some cases, the abdominal fetus dies and becomes calcified, forming a so-called stone fetus or lithopedion.

18. **A**   The blastocyst usually implants on the superior part of the posterior wall of the uterine cavity. Implantation occurs more often on the posterior than on the anterior wall. Implantation of the blastocyst outside of the uterine lumen (extra-uterine) is called an ectopic pregnancy.

19. **E**   Implantation of the blastocyst in the lower part of the uterine cervix in the region of the internal os may cover the entrance to the cervix, resulting in a condition known as placenta previa, in which the placenta may completely or partially cover the internal opening of the cervical canal. Serious hemorrhage may occur as a result of premature separation of the placenta during pregnancy or at delivery. For this reason, the fetus is delivered by cesarean section.

20. **D**   Ovarian pregnancy is relatively uncommon, with an incidence of approximately 0.5% of all ectopic pregnancies. In an ovarian pregnancy, fertilization of the oocyte probably occurs within the ovary, or in the ampulla of the uterine tube with subsequent implantation in the ovary after becoming dislodged from the tube. Because of intra-abdominal hemorrhage and other medical complications, surgical management is necessary.

Formation of Germ Layers and Early Tissue and Organ Differentiation

4

Objectives

Be able to:

- Describe the formation and growth of the primitive streak, using simple diagrams to illustrate formation of the intraembryonic mesoderm and the human embryo.
- Define primitive knot, primitive groove, and primitive pit.
- Trace the development of the notochord, using simple diagrammatic sections of 3-week embryos.
- Define notochordal process, notochordal canal, and notochordal plate.
- Give an account of the development of the neural tube, using simple sketches.
- Define neural plate, neural groove, neural folds, and neural crest.
- Illustrate, with simple sketches, the development of the following: somites, paraxial mesoderm, intermediate mesoderm, lateral mesoderm, intraembryonic coelom, tertiary villi, blood, and blood vessels.
- Construct and label diagrams showing the early development of the cardiovascular system and the sites of blood formation.
- Define angioblasts and blood islands.
- Write brief notes on the allantois, oropharyngeal membrane, and cloacal membrane.

■ FIVE-CHOICE COMPLETION QUESTIONS

Directions: Each of the following statements or questions is followed by five suggested responses or completions. **Select the one best answer** in each case.

1. Human chorionic gonadotropin (hCG) is a hormone produced by the
   - A. syncytiotrophoblast
   - B. anterior pituitary gland
   - C. corpus luteum of pregnancy
   - D. theca folliculi
   - E. hypophysis cerebri

2. The primitive streak first appears at the beginning of the _____ week.
   - A. first
   - B. second
   - C. third
   - D. fourth
   - E. fifth

Five-Choice Completion Questions *Continued*

3. The notochordal process lengthens by migration of cells from the
   A. notochord
   B. primitive streak
   C. notochordal plate
   D. primitive node
   E. neural plate

4. The notochordal plate infolds to form the
   A. neural tube
   B. neurenteric canal
   C. notochordal process
   D. notochordal canal
   E. notochord

5. During the third week, the neurenteric canal connects the amniotic cavity and the
   A. allantois
   B. neural tube
   C. caudal neuropore
   D. yolk sac
   E. chorionic cavity

6. The intraembryonic coelom located cranial to the oropharyngeal membrane becomes the
   A. mouth cavity
   B. stomodeum
   C. pericardial cavity
   D. pharyngeal cavity
   E. pleural cavity

7. The cloacal membrane consists of
   A. embryonic endoderm, mesoderm, and ectoderm
   B. a circular area of endoderm fused to embryonic mesoderm
   C. endoderm of the roof of the yolk sac and embryonic ectoderm
   D. the prechordal plate and the overlying embryonic ectoderm
   E. extraembryonic layers of the mesoderm

8. The specialized group of mesenchymal cells that aggregate to form blood islands are called
   A. hemoblasts
   B. angioblasts
   C. fibroblasts
   D. mesoblasts
   E. none of the above

9. The primitive blood cells of the 3-week embryo first begin to form
   A. at 19 to 20 days
   B. in the embryonic disc
   C. on the yolk sac
   D. in the liver
   E. on the allantois

10. A pregnant woman who has missed two menstrual periods wants to know her expected date of delivery. In practice, which of the following would you use?
    A. menstrual history
    B. date of coitus
    C. time of ovulation
    D. probable time of fertilization
    E. vaginal examination

11. A hydatidiform mole was diagnosed in a 30-year-old woman with a history of intermittent bleeding during the first trimester. This disorder is associated with all the following, *except:*
    A. embryonic death
    B. absence of tertiary villi
    C. decrease in hCG production
    D. potential for cancer
    E. cystic swelling of the chorionic villi

Five-Choice Completion Questions *Continued*

12. Ultrasonography revealed the presence of a sacrococcygeal teratoma in a near-term fetus. Which of the following is involved in this defect?
    A. persistence of the notochord
    B. primitive streak remnants
    C. prechordal plate
    D. extraembryonic mesoderm
    E. neural plate

13. Regarding the third week of development, which of the following is *incorrect*?
    A. The notochord induces formation of the neural tube
    B. Embryonic heart beat can be detected
    C. Somites begin to form
    D. Secondary villi become tertiary villi
    E. Heart tubes begin to fuse

14. The primitive streak
    A. extends from the primitive node to the oropharyngeal membrane
    B. is caudal to the notochord
    C. becomes the vertebral column
    D. is a thickening of endoderm
    E. induces the formation of the neural tube

15. The chromosomes of complete hydatidiform moles are
    A. always maternal in origin
    B. entirely of paternal origin
    C. always dispermic
    D. always monospermic
    E. both maternal and paternal in origin

■ ANSWERS AND EXPLANATIONS

1. **A** The syncytiotrophoblast layer of the trophoblast produces hCG, which stimulates the corpus luteum of pregnancy to increase in size and to continue producing hormones. Progesterone produced by the corpus luteum is necessary for maintenance of pregnancy during the early months. Thereafter, progesterone is produced by the syncytiotrophoblast of the placenta.

2. **C** The primitive streak usually appears in 15-day-old embryos (i.e., at the beginning of the third week). Cells from the primitive streak on the surface of the epiblast pass between the ectoderm and the endoderm and form the third germ layer (mesoderm).

3. **D** If you chose **B,** the primitive streak, you are partly right because the primitive node is the cranial end of the primitive streak. **D** is the better answer. Cells migrate cranially from the primitive node to form a midline cord known as the notochordal process. The primitive node is a thickening of the epiblast at the cranial end of the primitive streak. In addition to forming the notochordal process, cells from the primitive node also form intraembryonic mesoderm.

4. **E** The notochordal plate infolds to form the notochord. The primordium of the notochord is the notochordal process. The notochordal canal develops in the no-

Answers and Explanations *Continued*

tochordal process as the primitive pit invaginates into it.

5. **D** The neurenteric canal is associated with late stages of notochord development. It represents the part of the notochordal canal that does not disappear when the floor of the notochordal process degenerates. The neurenteric canal connects the amniotic cavity and the yolk sac. It usually disappears when the notochord is fully developed (about 5 weeks). In most cases, the brief existence of the canal is of no significance.

6. **C** The pericardial cavity and the developing heart are carried ventrally within the head fold as the brain grows rapidly during the fourth week. The pericardial cavity forms by confluence of small, isolated spaces in the cardiogenic (heart-forming) mesoderm, which lies cranial to the oropharyngeal membrane.

7. **C** The cloacal membrane is the circular bilaminar area where the embryonic endoderm of the roof of the yolk sac contacts and fuses with the overlying embryonic ectoderm caudal to the primitive streak. There is no mesoderm between the two layers composing the cloacal membrane. The area where the prechordal plate fuses with the overlying ectoderm is called the oropharyngeal membrane.

8. **B** Angioblasts are specialized mesenchymal cells that give rise to blood and to the vascular and lymphatic systems. Fibroblasts are connective tissue cells that form fibrous tissues in the body. Hemoblasts are blood cells that usually are called hemocytoblasts.

9. **C** Primitive blood first forms in the extraembryonic mesoderm associated with the yolk sac at 15 to 16 days. Later it forms in the allantois and connecting stalk. Blood formation does not begin in the embryo until the sixth week, when it

forms in the liver. Hence, the blood in the 3-week embryo forms in the extraembryonic membranes and flows into the cardiovascular system as the embryonic vessels form.

10. **A** In practice, the age of the embryo is calculated from the first day of the last menstrual period because this information usually is readily available. The most accurate estimation of the date of delivery is from the time of fertilization because the ovum usually is fertilized within 12 hours after ovulation. Clinical signs of pregnancy may be evident by vaginal examination by about the sixth week because of an increase in uterine size and softening of the cervix. The fundus of the uterus can be palpated from the abdominal wall by the third month. Ultrasonography is commonly used for estimating embryonic and fetal age.

11. **C** A hydatidiform mole results from abnormal proliferation of the trophoblast even though the embryo is no longer alive. The chorionic villi do not become vascularized to form tertiary villi and soon degenerate to form a large mass of cystic swellings. The excessive trophoblast produces large amounts of hCG. About 2% of these moles develop into malignant lesions called choriocarcinomas, which typically metastasize to various parts of the body (e.g., the lungs, liver, vagina, and brain).

12. **B** The primitive streak forms intraembryonic mesoderm until the end of the fourth week, after which it slowly regresses and disappears. Persistence of primitive streak cells gives rise to a tumor known as a teratoma in the region of the sacrum and coccyx. These tumors are more common in females than in males and may become cancerous during infancy. Because of the pleuripotent nature of the primitive streak cells, many tumors contain different types of tissue.

Answers and Explanations *Continued*

13. **B** Paired, longitudinal, endothelium-lined heart tubes develop from mesenchymal cells in the cardiogenic area. During the third week, the two heart tubes fuse to form a single primitive heart tube. By the end of the third week, the primitive heart is beating and blood is circulating through a primitive cardiovascular system. Embryonic heart beat can be detected ultrasonographically during the fifth week. Somites begin to form before the end of the third week, and 42 to 44 pairs of somites are present by the end of the fifth week. The notochord induces neural tube formation during the third week, and neural tube formation is completed during the fourth week. By the end of the third week, blood vessels develop from the mesenchymal tissue in the core of the secondary villi, transforming them into tertiary villi.

14. **B** The primitive streak appears at the beginning of the third week, and it is derived from epiblast cells. The primitive streak contributes to the formation of intraembryonic mesoderm and the notochord. By the beginning of the fifth week, the primitive streak degenerates and normally disappears. Remnants of the primitive streak may persist and give rise to a sacrococcygeal teratoma, one of the most common tumors in the neonate. The primitive streak is located caudal to the notochord, which is involved in the induction of the neural tube.

15. **B** On the basis of karyotype and other characteristic histopathologic features, hydatidiform moles are classified as either complete or partial. The chromosomes of complete hydatidiform moles are entirely of paternal origin. More than 90% of complete hydatidiform moles are monospermic, resulting from the fertilization of an empty oocyte by a haploid sperm followed by duplication. A dispermic mole results from the fertilization of an empty oocyte by two sperms. The risk of a complete or partial mole increases after spontaneous abortion, and in some cases a molar pregnancy may lead to a trophoblastic tumor, that is, choriocarcinoma.

■ FIVE-CHOICE ASSOCIATION QUESTIONS

Directions: Each group of questions below consists of a numbered list of descriptive words or phrases accompanied by a diagram with certain parts indicated by letters and a list of lettered headings. For each numbered word or phrase, **select the lettered part or heading** that matches it correctly and then insert the letter in the space to the right of the appropriate number. Sometimes more than one numbered word or phrase may be correctly matched to the same lettered part or heading.

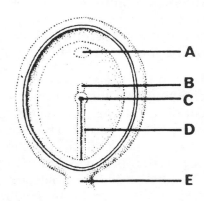

A. Allantois
B. Primitive streak
C. Notochord
D. Blood island
E. Neural plate

1. _____ Notochordal process
2. _____ Site of the prechordal plate
3. _____ Gives rise to mesoderm
4. _____ Ventral layer of the oropharyngeal membrane
5. _____ Primitive pit
6. _____ Aggregation of angioblasts
7. _____ Diverticulum of the yolk sac
8. _____ Induces embryonic ectoderm to thicken
9. _____ Forms the basis of the axial skeleton
10. _____ Gives rise to the brain and spinal cord
11. _____ Source of mesenchyme
12. _____ Rudimentary structure
13. _____ Appears in extraembryonic membranes

14. _____ Wall of the amniotic sac
15. _____ Neural groove
16. _____ Derived from the primitive streak
17. _____ Embryonic ectoderm

18. _____ Derived from paraxial mesoderm
19. _____ Derived from the notochordal process
20. _____ Gives rise to an adult body cavity
21. _____ Splanchnopleure
22. _____ Fusing to form the neural tube

Five-Choice Association Questions *Continued*

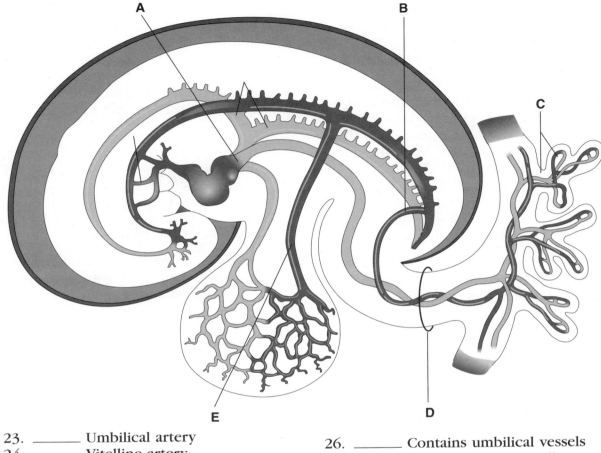

23. _____ Umbilical artery
24. _____ Vitelline artery
25. _____ Sinus venosus

26. _____ Contains umbilical vessels
27. _____ Tertiary chorionic villus

■ ANSWERS AND EXPLANATIONS

1. **B** The notochordal process is a rod-shaped structure composed of cells derived from the primitive node. It is the primordium of the notochord, a cellular structure that defines the primordial axis of the embryo.

2. **A** The site of the prechordal plate is indicated in the drawing by a dotted oval to indicate that it is not visible from the dorsal surface of the embryonic disc. The prechordal plate is a circular area of thickened embryonic endoderm in the cranial part of the roof of the yolk sac. The prechordal plate, together with the overlying embryonic ectoderm, later constitutes the oropharyngeal membrane.

3. **D** The primitive streak, a linear band, gives rise to mesoderm mainly during the third week. As the mesoderm is produced by the primitive streak, it extends laterally until it becomes continuous with the extraembryonic mesoderm on the amnion and yolk sac. The intraembryonic mesoderm thickens on each side of the embryonic axis to form two longitudinal columns of paraxial mesoderm.

4. **A** The ventral layer of the bilaminar oropharyngeal membrane is the prechordal

Answers and Explanations *Continued*

plate; the dorsal layer is embryonic ecto-derm. This membrane ruptures during the fourth week, bringing the primitive oral cavity into communication with the primordial pharynx.

5. **C** The primitive pit is a depression in the primitive node at the cranial end of the primitive streak. It extends into the notochordal process and forms the noto-chordal canal. Thus, it is the entrance to the notochordal canal. It later forms the opening of the neurenteric canal, which temporarily connects the amniotic cavity with the yolk sac.

6. **D** Mesenchymal cells known as angioblasts aggregate to form isolated masses and cords called blood islands. These masses give rise to primordial plasma, blood cells, and blood vessels. Blood islands form first in the yolk sac, chorion, allantois, and connecting stalk, but they develop in the embryo about 2 days later.

7. **A** The allantois is a vestigial structure that later becomes the urachus (median umbilical ligament). It serves as a reservoir for excretory products in some species, but it is nonfunctional in human embryos. Later, its blood vessels become the umbilical vessels.

8. **C** The developing notochord and the adjacent paraxial mesoderm are thought to produce inductive substances that stimulate development of the neural plate from the overlying embryonic ectoderm.

9. **C** The notochord forms the basis of the axial skeleton. The vertebrae develop around it, and then it degenerates. In between the vertebrae, the notochord gives rise to the nucleus pulposus of the intervertebral disc.

10. **E** The neural plate is a thickened area of ectoderm (neuroectoderm) that over-lies and extends on each side of the noto-chord. The neural plate invaginates to form a neural groove. In later develop-ment, the neural folds meet dorsally to

form the neural tube. The cranial part of the neural tube gives rise to the brain, and the larger remaining part forms the spinal cord. The notochord and paraxial mesoderm produce inductive substances that stimulate or induce the overlying ec-toderm to thicken and form the neural plate.

11. **B** The primitive streak produces meso-derm, which gives rise to mesenchyme (embryonic connective tissue). Mesen-chyme forms a packing tissue around de-veloping organs and gives rise to connec-tive tissues and muscles.

12. **A** The allantois is a rudimentary struc-ture. Although the allantois does not func-tion in human embryos, it is important because blood formation occurs in its walls and its blood vessels become the umbilical vessels.

13. **D** The blood islands first appear in the walls of the yolk sac, the allantois, and the connecting stalk. These extraembry-onic membranes are derived from the zy-gote, but they are not part of the em-bryo. The roof of the yolk sac becomes incorporated into the embryo during the fourth week and forms the primordial gut. Blood islands form in the embryo about 2 days after they appear on the yolk sac.

14. **C** The amnion encloses the amniotic cavity, forming an amniotic sac. It con-tains fluid that bathes the embryonic disc, forming its floor. The wall of this sac consists of an inner epithelial layer of cells covered externally by extraembry-onic somatic mesoderm.

15. **A** The neural groove forms as the neu-ral plate invaginates to form a neural fold on each side. The folds later fuse to form the neural tube, the primordium of the central nervous system (brain and spinal cord). The ectoderm lateral to the folds, known as surface ectoderm, gives rise to the epidermis of the skin.

16. **E** The intraembryonic mesoderm is de-rived from the primitive streak. The prim-

Answers and Explanations *Continued*

itive streak produces mesoderm rapidly during the third and fourth weeks.

17. **B** The embryonic ectoderm in the region indicated forms a neural fold. The neural folds soon fuse, converting the neural plate into the neural tube, the primordium of the central nervous system (brain and spinal cord).

18. **C** The somites are paired cubical masses derived by division or segmentation of the paraxial mesoderm. The first pair of somites is formed a short distance caudal to the tip of the notochord, and successive somites are progressively formed from paraxial mesoderm. Most somites appear between days 20 and 30; they give rise to the axial skeleton and its associated musculature.

19. **E** The notochord arises from the notochordal process. The notochord is a cellular rod that defines the primordial axis of the embryo. Mesenchymal cells from the somites later surround it and give rise to the mesenchymal bodies of the vertebrae. The notochord within the developing vertebrae later degenerates.

20. **A** The intraembryonic coelom in the area indicated gives rise to part of the peritoneal cavity. The coelom appears here as a space within the lateral mesoderm, splitting it into somatic and splanchnic layers. The transverse section is cut through the caudal region of the lateral extensions of the horseshoe-shaped body cavity or coelom.

21. **D** The embryonic splanchnopleure is composed of splanchnic mesoderm and endoderm and represents the future wall of the primordial gut. The endoderm gives rise to the epithelium and glands of the digestive tract; the mesoderm gives rise to its muscular and fibrous elements.

22. **B** The neural folds are fusing to form the neural tube, the primordium of the

brain and spinal cord. These folds form as the neural plate invaginates along its central axis to form a neural groove with neural folds on each side.

23. **B** The paired umbilical arteries are branches of the dorsal aortae. They transport partially deoxygenated blood and waste products from the embryo to the chorionic villi of the placenta.

24. **E** The vitelline arteries are branches of the dorsal aortae to the yolk sac. The vitelline arteries and the vitelline veins are in communication through a vascular plexus on the yolk sac.

25. **A** Blood enters the sinus venosus from the embryo via the cardinal veins, from the developing placenta via the umbilical vein, and from the yolk sac via the vitelline veins. Blood from the sinus venosus enters the primordial heart.

26. **D** The umbilical cord develops from the connecting stalk. It contains the paired umbilical arteries and the umbilical vein. The umbilical cord is the vital connection between the embryo and the placenta because the umbilical vessels transport gases, nutrients, essential substances, and waste products.

27. **C** By the end of the third week, blood vessels differentiate from mesenchymal cells present in the core of the secondary villi to form the tertiary chorionic villi. The blood vessels in the tertiary villi soon become connected with the primordial heart via blood vessels that differentiate in the mesenchyme of the chorion and connecting stalk. A primordial embryonic circulation is established by the end of the third week. Oxygen and nutrients in the maternal blood in the intervillous spaces diffuse through the walls of the villi and enter the embryo's blood. Carbon dioxide and waste products diffuse from fetal blood through the walls of the villi into the maternal blood.

Organogenetic Period: The Fourth to Eighth Weeks

5

Objectives

Be able to:

- Draw and label simple sketches showing the main developmental events of each week during the organogenetic period.
- Explain why the fourth to eighth weeks constitute a critical period of human development.
- Define neuropore, pharyngeal arch, aortic arch, otic pit, lens placode, limb bud, and cervical flexure.
- Estimate the age of embryos traced from drawings in your textbook, using the table in your textbook and crown-rump measurements.
- Briefly indicate what each germ layer normally contributes to the tissues and organs of the embryo.
- Discuss induction, using the neural plate and the eye as examples.
- Discuss the establishment of general body form resulting from folding of the embryo, with special reference to the effect of this process on the septum transversum, heart, foregut, midgut, allantois, and yolk sac.

■ FIVE-CHOICE COMPLETION QUESTIONS

Directions: Each of the following statements or questions is followed by five suggested responses or completions. **Select the one best answer** in each case.

1. All the essential features of external body form of the embryo are completed by the end of the _____ week.
   - A. 4th
   - B. 6th
   - C. 8th
   - D. 10th
   - E. 12th

2. During the early part of the fourth week, the rate of growth at the periphery of the embryonic disc fails to keep pace with the rate of growth of the
   - A. yolk sac
   - B. amniotic cavity
   - C. embryonic coelom
   - D. notochordal process
   - E. neural tube

Five-Choice Completion Questions *Continued*

3. By the middle of the fourth week, the neural folds at the cranial end of the embryo have begun to develop into the
   A. neural crest
   B. spinal cord
   C. brain
   D. neural groove
   E. neural tube

4. After folding of the head region, the mesodermal structure lying just caudal to the pericardial cavity is the
   A. developing heart
   B. connecting stalk
   C. primitive streak
   D. septum transversum
   E. notochord

5. Each of the following structures turns onto the ventral surface of the embryo during folding of the head, *except* the
   A. oropharyngeal membrane
   B. notochord
   C. heart
   D. pericardial cavity
   E. septum transversum

6. The terminal dilated part of the hindgut is called the
   A. allantois
   B. yolk stalk
   C. cloaca
   D. vitelline duct
   E. cecum

7. Each of the following structures is derived from mesoderm, *except:*
   A. muscle
   B. cartilage
   C. mesenchyme
   D. blood vessel
   E. epidermis

8. Which of the following structures is believed to be a primary inductor during organogenesis?
   A. somite
   B. notochord
   C. yolk sac
   D. primitive streak
   E. lens

9. Each of the following is a distinctive characteristic of 4-week-old embryos, *except:*
   A. somites
   B. hand plates
   C. pharyngeal arches
   D. lower limb buds
   E. neuropores

10. The most frequently used method for measuring the length of 5-week-old embryos is
    A. greatest length
    B. standing height
    C. crown-rump length
    D. crown-heel length
    E. total length

11. The age of the embryo illustrated below is _____ weeks.

    A. 3
    B. 4
    C. 5
    D. 6
    E. 7

Five-Choice Completion Questions *Continued*

12. A pathologic examination of an aborted embryo revealed that the embryo was about 20 mm in length, with the midgut herniated into the proximal part of the umbilical cord. The trunk of the embryo was elongated and straightened. Nipples were present, and the cerebral vesicles were prominent. Digital rays of the hand and foot plates were also evident. Which of the following is likely to be the approximate age of the embryo?

   A. 4 weeks   D. 7 weeks
   B. 5 weeks   E. 8 weeks
   C. 6 weeks

13. Characteristics of embryos early in the eighth week include

   A. webbed fingers
   B. eyelids
   C. umbilical herniation
   D. short tail
   E. all of the above

14. Each of the following structures is derived from the neural crest *except:*

   A. pigment cells   D. pharyngeal arch cartilages
   B. bulbar and conal ridges in the heart   E. medulla of the suprarenal gland
   C. pineal body

■ ANSWERS AND EXPLANATIONS

1. **C** By the end of the embryonic period (8 weeks), the beginnings of all major external and internal structures have developed. Because of this, these 5 weeks constitute the most critical period of development and the time when major developmental anomalies may occur.

2. **E** Because of the rapid growth of the neural tube, the embryo bulges into the amniotic cavity and the head and tail regions fold under the cranial and caudal parts of the embryonic disc. Concurrently, marked folding occurs along the lateral margins of the disc.

3. **C** By the middle of the fourth week, the neural folds at the center of the embryo have started to move together and fuse into the neural tube. At the cranial end of the embryo, the thick neural folds indicate where the brain will develop. By the end of the fourth week, the neural folds in the cranial region have fused to form primary brain vesicles, which develop into the brain.

4. **D** The mesodermal mass known as the septum transversum forms the caudal wall of the pericardial cavity. This mesodermal septum is the primordium of the central tendon of the diaphragm. After folding of the head, the heart lies dorsal to the pericardial cavity. The primitive streak and the connecting stalk lie considerably caudal to the pericardial cavity.

5. **B** The cranial end of the notochord may bend slightly as the forebrain folds ven-

Answers and Explanations *Continued*

trally, but the notochord does not turn onto the ventral surface as the other structures do (e.g., the heart).

6. **C** Shortly after the caudal part of the yolk sac is incorporated into the embryo as the hindgut, the terminal part of the hindgut dilates to form the cloaca. Its cavity is separated from the amniotic cavity by the cloacal membrane.

7. **E** The epidermis is derived from the surface ectoderm. The dermis of the skin is derived from mesoderm, as are all types of connective tissue. The cartilages in the pharyngeal arches are derived from neural crest cells.

8. **B** From experiments on lower vertebrates, it is well established that substances produced by the notochordal process and later the notochord induce the neural plate to form. The lenses appear to function as secondary inductors.

9. **B** Hand plates are not visible during the fourth week. They are not distinctive characteristics of the limbs until the fifth week.

10. **C** Crown-rump measurements are most commonly taken. Greatest length is used for straight embryos (e.g., during the third week). Crown-heel measurements (standing height) are sometimes used for older embryos, but they often are difficult to make on formalin-fixed embryos

because these are difficult to straighten. Ultrasound measurements are used to determine the age of embryos in utero.

11. **B** The distinctive characteristics of the 4-week embryo (about 28 days) shown here are (1) four pharyngeal arches, (2) a flipper-like upper limb bud, and (3) a small lower limb bud.

12. **D** The embryo is about 7 weeks old. Umbilical herniation is usually obvious during this period. Before the seventh week, the embryo is somewhat curved with hand and foot plates. After the seventh week, notches appear between the digital rays and the digits are formed. By the seventh week, the nipples and the prominent cerebral vesicles are evident.

13. **E** Webbed fingers and notches between the digits of the feet are characteristic features of embryos during the early part of the eighth week. The presence of eyelids, a short tail, and the umbilical herniation are also features of the early part of this week.

14. **C** Neuroectodermal cells become segregated to form the neural crest following fusion of the neural folds and formation of the neural tube. The pineal body is derived from the neural tube (brain). Pigment cells, the medulla of the suprarenal gland, pharyngeal arch cartilages, bulbar and conal ridges in the heart, as well as other structures, develop from neural crest cells.

■ FIVE-CHOICE ASSOCIATION QUESTIONS

Directions: Each group of questions below consists of a numbered list of descriptive words or phrases accompanied by a diagram with certain parts indicated by letters or by a list of lettered headings. For each numbered word or phrase, **select the letter or heading** that matches it correctly. Then insert the letter in the space to the right of the appropriate number. Sometimes more than one numbered word or phrase may be correctly matched to the same lettered part or heading.

Five-Choice Association Questions *Continued*

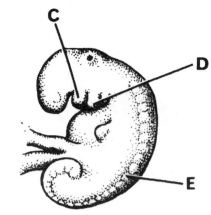

1. _____ Hyoid arch
2. _____ Gives rise to the mandible
3. _____ Forms from paraxial mesoderm

A. Limb bud
B. Neuropore
C. Septum transversum
D. Cervical sinus
E. Stomodeum

4. _____ First branchial pharyngeal arch
5. _____ Neuropore
6. _____ Optic sulcus in neural fold

7. _____ Forms major part of the diaphragm
8. _____ Primordial mouth
9. _____ Outgrowth of the body wall
10. _____ Forms as a result of the head fold
11. _____ Closes during the fourth week
12. _____ Ectodermal depression in the neck

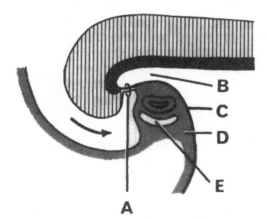

A. fourth week
B. fifth week
C. sixth week
D. seventh week
E. eighth week

13. _____ Septum transversum
14. _____ Part of the embryonic coelom
15. _____ Oropharyngeal membrane
16. _____ Separates the amniotic cavity from the foregut
17. _____ Gives rise to a major part of the diaphragm

18. _____ Lens placodes recognizable
19. _____ Umbilical herniation noticeable
20. _____ Retinal pigment first recognizable
21. _____ Lower limb buds appear
22. _____ Embryo essentially straight
23. _____ Cervical sinuses visible
24. _____ Tail disappears

Five-Choice Association Questions *Continued*

25. _____ Cloaca
26. _____ Produces embryonic mesoderm
27. _____ Separates the amniotic cavity from the hindgut
28. _____ Vestigial structure
29. _____ Amnion
30. _____ Site of blood formation in the early embryo

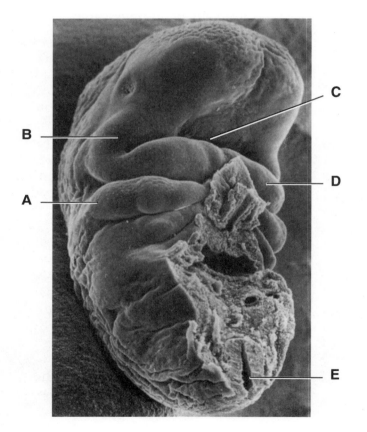

31. _____ Second pharyngeal (branchial) arch
32. _____ Derived from neural tube
33. _____ Stomodeum
34. _____ Will form the lower jaw
35. _____ Gives rise to upper jaw
36. _____ Defect in formation results in a severe type of spina bifida

■ ANSWERS AND EXPLANATIONS

1. **D** The second or hyoid pharyngeal arch is recognizable early in the fourth week. As its name implies, this arch gives rise to part of the hyoid bone. Mesenchyme in this arch also gives rise to the muscles of facial expression and to various skeletal structures.

2. **C** The mandibular prominences of the first pair of pharyngeal arches give rise to the lower jaw or mandible. Rostral extensions of the first arch, called maxillary prominences, give rise to the upper jaw or maxilla.

3. **E** The somites form by differentiation and division of the longitudinal columns of paraxial mesoderm into cubical segments. The somites give rise to most of the axial skeleton, the associated musculature, and the dermis of the skin.

4. **C** The pointer indicates the mandibular prominence of the first pharyngeal arch. The mandibular prominences merge with each other during the fourth week and give rise to the mandible, lower lip, and inferior part of the face.

5. **B** The caudal neuropore is indicated. This structure is also referred to as the posterior neuropore. It is better to call it the caudal neuropore because it is always at the caudal end of the embryo. The neuropores (rostral and caudal) normally are closed by the end of the fourth week. The rostral neuropore closes on day 25 or 26, and the caudal neuropore usually closes about 2 days later. Defective closure of the caudal neuropore gives rise to a severe anomaly called spina bifida.

6. **A** The pointer indicates the optic sulcus in a neural fold. This sulcus is the primordium of the optic vesicle, an outgrowth of the forebrain vesicle.

7. **C** The septum transversum is a mass of mesoderm that first appears cranial to the developing heart. After folding of the embryo, it lies caudal to the heart, where it forms part of the primordial diaphragm. Later it develops into the central tendon of the diaphragm.

8. **E** The stomodeum or primordial mouth cavity is an ectodermal depression that develops during the fourth week as the head folds. Initially, it is separated from the primordial pharynx (cranial part of the foregut) by the oropharyngeal membrane. By the end of the fourth week, this membrane ruptures, bringing the mouth cavity into communication with the foregut.

9. **A** The limb buds form on the ventrolateral body wall during the fourth week. The upper limb buds usually appear on day 26, and the lower limb buds are visible about 2 days later.

10. **E** The stomodeum (primordial mouth cavity) and the foregut form as the head folds ventrally. The cranial part of the yolk sac is incorporated into the embryo during this longitudinal folding. At first, the stomodeum and the foregut are separate cavities, but they become continuous during the fourth week when the oropharyngeal membrane ruptures.

11. **B** The neuropores close during the fourth week. The rostral neuropore closes on day 25 or 26, and the caudal neuropore closes about 2 days later. Defects of closure of the neuropores give rise to congenital anomalies of the central nervous system (e.g., spina bifida).

12. **D** The cervical sinus is a depression in the surface ectoderm on each side of the future neck. It forms when the second pharyngeal arch overgrows the third and fourth arches. The second and third arches come to lie at the bottom of a pit called the cervical sinus. It is visible externally only during the fifth week.

Answers and Explanations *Continued*

13. **D**   The septum transversum is a mass of mesoderm that is first recognizable cranial to the pericardial coelom. After folding, it lies caudal to the heart and pericardial coelom. The septum transversum gives rise to the central tendon of the diaphragm.

14. **E**   The pericardial coelom is the part of the embryonic coelom that gives rise to the pericardial cavity. It first appears in the cardiogenic mesoderm, where it lies cranial to the oropharyngeal membrane. After folding, the pericardial coelom lies ventral to the developing heart, as shown in the drawing.

15. **A**   The oropharyngeal membrane develops during the third week as the prechordal plate fuses with the overlying embryonic ectoderm. This membrane ruptures during the fourth week.

16. **A**   The oropharyngeal membrane separates the amniotic cavity from the foregut (primordial pharynx). Amniotic fluid may enter the primordial mouth or stomodeum, but it cannot pass into the primordial pharynx until the oropharyngeal membrane ruptures.

17. **D**   The septum transversum is the first recognizable part of the developing diaphragm. It appears cranially at the end of the third week, when the pericardial coelom forms. The septum transversum later forms the central tendon of the diaphragm.

18. **A**   The lens placodes are recognizable during the fourth week as thickenings of the surface ectoderm. They give rise to the lens vesicles, the primordia of the lenses of the eyes.

19. **D**   As the midgut loop develops, it herniates into the umbilical cord because there is not enough room for it in the abdomen. This physiologic process or herniation begins during the fifth week, but the intestines do not usually form a noticeable swelling of the cord until the seventh week.

20. **B**   Pigment appears in the retinae of the eyes during the fifth week, making the eyes more obvious. Eye development is first evident early in the fourth week, when the optic sulci develop.

21. **A**   The lower limb buds appear toward the end of the fourth week as ventrolateral swellings of the body walls. Each bud consists of a mass of mesenchyme that is covered by surface ectoderm. The upper limb buds form around the middle of the fourth week.

22. **A**   The embryo is essentially straight during the early part of the fourth week. Near the middle of the fourth week, the embryo begins to fold in the longitudinal and horizontal planes, giving the embryo a characteristic C-shaped curvature.

23. **B**   The cervical sinuses are visible externally during the fifth week. The external openings of these sinuses usually close by the end of the fifth week. Remnants of parts of the cervical sinuses may give rise to anomalies called branchial or lateral cervical cysts.

24. **E**   The tail often is visible during the early part of the eighth week, but it disappears by the end of the eighth week.

25. **B**   The cloaca is the dilated caudal portion of the hindgut; the allantois enters it ventrally. The cloaca is separated from the amniotic cavity by the cloacal membrane.

26. **C**   The primitive streak appears during the early part of the third week and produces mesoderm rapidly until the end of the fourth week. Thereafter, mesoderm production from this source slows down.

27. **E**   The cloacal membrane separates the amniotic cavity from the cloacal region

Answers and Explanations *Continued*

of the hindgut. This membrane consists of fused layers of embryonic ectoderm and endoderm. It is later divided into anal and urogenital membranes during the seventh week; these membranes soon rupture.

28. **A**   The allantois is a rudimentary, vestigial structure that forms during the third week as a diverticulum of the caudal wall of the yolk sac. It remains very small and gives rise to the urachus, a tubular structure that runs from the urinary bladder to the umbilicus. Its adult derivative is the median umbilical ligament.

29. **D**   The amnion forms during the second week. It is attached to the margins of the embryonic disc and forms the wall of the amniotic sac.

30. **A**   Blood begins to form in the mesenchyme around the allantois and yolk sac during the third week. These are the only sites of blood formation until blood begins to form in the liver during the sixth week.

31. **A**   Five pharyngeal (branchial) arches are formed in the embryo. The second pharyngeal arch appears at the beginning of the fourth week. The embryo is about 32 days old with four pairs of pharyngeal arches; the fourth pharyngeal arch is smaller and not clearly delineated. The second pharyngeal arch overgrows the third and fourth arches, forming a transitory ectoderm-lined cervical sinus that becomes obliterated.

32. **E**   The neural tube is formed following fusion of the neural folds by the end of the fourth week. It gives rise to the brain and spinal cord (E). Spina bifida, an anomaly of the spinal cord and the overlying vertebrae, results from a defect in the fusion of the neural folds.

33. **C**   An ectoderm-lined depression, known as the stomodeum, partly contributes to the formation of the oral cavity. It is located at the cranial end of the embryo, bounded by the maxillary and mandibular prominences. At the floor of the stomodeum is the oropharyngeal membrane, which separates the stomodeum from the primordial pharynx. The oropharyngeal membrane breaks down at about 26 days, bringing the primordial pharynx (part of the digestive tract) into communication with the amniotic cavity.

34. **D**   The first pharyngeal arch gives rise to both the maxillary and mandibular prominences. The lower jaw is formed from the larger mandibular prominences, which are paired at first, but the medial ends merge and fuse during the fourth week. The lower jaw and the lower lip are the first parts of the face to develop.

35. **B**   The shorter and smaller maxillary prominences form the lateral boundaries of the stomodeum. The maxillary prominences, which lie just below the overhanging frontonasal prominence (forebrain), grow medially and merge with the medial nasal prominences to form the upper lip. The upper jaw develops from the maxillary prominences, which also give rise to several facial and cranial bones.

36. **E**   Fusion of the neural folds occurs during the fourth week, forming the neural tube. The neural tube gives rise to the brain and spinal cord. The rostral neuropore closes on day 25 or 26, and the caudal neuropore closes about 2 days later. Neural tube anomalies, including spina bifida, occur as a result of defects in closure of the neural tube.

Fetal Period 6

Objectives

Be able to:

- State the significant differences between development during the embryonic and fetal periods, and comment on differences in the vulnerability of embryos and fetuses to teratogenic agents.
- Discuss the effects of inadequate uterine environment, indicating the possible effects of environmental agents (e.g., viruses) and other factors on fetal growth and development.
- Describe the differences between fetuses that are of low birth weight because of intrauterine growth retardation and those that are premature.
- Write brief notes on the following techniques used for assessing the status of the human fetus before birth: amniocentesis, fetoscopy, fetal blood sampling, chorionic villus sampling, and ultrasonography.

■ FIVE-CHOICE COMPLETION QUESTIONS

Directions: Each of the following statements or questions is followed by five suggested responses or completions. **Select the one best answer** in each case.

1. The head constitutes almost half the fetus at the beginning of the
   - A. 12th week
   - B. second trimester
   - C. fetal period
   - D. stage of quickening
   - E. embryonic period

2. The usual measurement for estimating fetal age is
   - A. crown-rump length
   - B. foot length
   - C. crown-heel length
   - D. leg length
   - E. head size

3. Which of the following statements about fetal age and weight seems to be closest to the normal relationship?
   - A. 8 weeks—10 gm
   - B. 12 weeks—200 gm
   - C. 20 weeks—800 gm
   - D. 26 weeks—1000 gm
   - E. 38 weeks—4400 gm

4. The fetal period begins
   - A. after all organs have completely developed
   - B. when the genitalia have distinctive characteristics
   - C. at the beginning of the ninth week
   - D. at the end of the first trimester
   - E. when the developing human is viable

Five-Choice Completion Questions *Continued*

5. Sexing of fetuses is first possible from examination of the external genitalia during the _____ week.
   - A. 8th
   - B. 9th
   - C. 10th
   - D. 11th
   - E. 12th

6. A fetus has a reasonable chance of surviving, if born prematurely, when its fertilization age is _____ weeks.
   - A. 12
   - B. 16
   - C. 18
   - D. 20
   - E. 24

7. Quickening, the period when fetal movements commonly are felt by the mother, usually occurs
   - A. near the end of the first trimester
   - B. around the middle of the second trimester
   - C. at the end of the second trimester
   - D. when the fetus becomes viable
   - E. during the so-called finishing period

8. The most likely cause of very low birth weight in full-term fetuses is
   - A. maternal malnutrition
   - B. prematurity
   - C. smoking
   - D. placental insufficiency
   - E. alcoholism

9. Amniocentesis commonly is used to
   - A. diagnose the chromosomal sex of fetuses
   - B. detect placental insufficiency
   - C. assess the degree of erythroblastosis fetalis
   - D. determine the composition of the amniotic fluid
   - E. determine the age of the fetus

10. Which of the following ultrasonographic measurements is most reliable for estimating fetal age?
    - A. crown-rump length
    - B. biparietal diameter of the head
    - C. dimension of the trunk
    - D. foot length
    - E. cheek to cheek

11. The age of a fetus was estimated from measurements of its crown-rump length using ultrasonography. How early can the sex of the fetus be clearly determined from the appearance of its external genitalia?
    - A. 9 weeks
    - B. 10 weeks
    - C. 12 weeks
    - D. 14 weeks
    - E. 16 weeks

12. Primary ossification centers first appear in the fetus after
    - A. 9 weeks
    - B. 13 weeks
    - C. 17 weeks
    - D. 21 weeks
    - E. 25 weeks

Five-Choice Completion Questions *Continued*

13. A woman who is about 8 weeks pregnant asked her doctor when she should begin to feel her "baby" moving. Your reply should be, at about
    A. 10 weeks
    B. 15 weeks
    C. 20 weeks
    D. 25 weeks
    E. 30 weeks

14. Oligohydramnios was diagnosed in a pregnant woman. This condition has been associated with one or more of the following *except:*
    A. decreased amniotic fluid volume
    B. placental insufficiency
    C. fetal renal disease
    D. esophageal atresia
    E. preterm rupture of the amniochorionic membrane

15. In a pregnancy that was medically terminated, a nonviable male fetus was recovered. The fetus had a crown-rump (CR) length of between 140 and 160 mm. The skin was covered with vernix caseosa. Fingernails and toenails were not present, and the eyes were closed. This fetus is about _____ weeks old.
    A. 14
    B. 18
    C. 22
    D. 28
    E. 32

16. An infant born after a prolonged pregnancy showed signs of the postmaturity syndrome. This often includes the following characteristic features *except:*
    A. thin appearance
    B. dry parchment-like skin
    C. decreased or absent vernix caseosa
    D. abundant lanugo hair
    E. long fingernails

■ ANSWERS AND EXPLANATIONS

1. **C** At 9 weeks, when the fetal period begins, the head constitutes almost half the fetus. Thereafter, growth of the head slows down compared with the rest of the body. By the end of the 12th week, the head represents almost one third of the length of the fetus. The stage of quickening, or the time when the fetal movements are recognized by the mother, does not occur until the 17- to 20-week period. By this stage, the head represents a little more than one quarter of the length of the fetus.

2. **A** Crown-rump measurements are the most useful criteria for estimating fetal age. The length of fetuses, like those of infants and children, varies considerably for a given age. Crown-heel measurements often are used for older fetuses, but they are less useful because of the difficulty in straightening the fetus. Foot length correlates well with length and is particularly useful for estimating the age of incomplete or macerated fetuses. Head size is used to estimate the age of mature fetuses (e.g., after 22 weeks).

3. **D** Most fetuses of 26 weeks weigh about 1000 gm and survive if born prematurely. Although there is no sharp limit of

Answers and Explanations *Continued*

development, age, or weight at which a fetus becomes viable, most fetuses that are younger or weigh less do not survive. All the other weights listed are high for the ages given. For example, 8-week fetuses usually weigh about 5 gm. Full-term fetuses (38 weeks after fertilization) may weigh 4400 gm, but this is heavy. The average weight of newborn infants is 3400 gm. Heavier women usually produce heavier infants, and underweight women usually have lighter infants. There is an increased frequency of low birth weights among teenage mothers, largely because they are still growing and so have greater nutritional requirements than do older women (i.e., young mothers may compete with their fetuses for nutrients).

4. **C** The fetal period begins at the beginning of the ninth week (i.e., during the first trimester). Most organs have mainly completed their development when the fetal period begins. The external genitalia do not acquire distinctive sexual characteristics until the end of the ninth week, and their mature form is not established until the 12th week. The intestines do not enter the abdomen until the 10th week, about 1 week after the beginning of the fetal period.

5. **C** The external genitalia of male and female fetuses appear somewhat similar until the end of the 12th week, but most people could identify the sex of 10-week embryos. The external genitalia are fully formed by the 12th week.

6. **E** Fetuses that weigh less than 1000 gm and are less than 24 weeks of age do not usually survive if born prematurely because of the immaturity of their respiratory systems. By 26 to 28 weeks, sufficient terminal air sacs, surfactant, and vascularity have formed for adequate gas exchange and maintenance of life.

7. **B** Fetal movements normally are felt by the mother around the middle of the sec-

ond trimester of pregnancy (17 to 20 weeks). Mothers who have been pregnant three or more times (multigravida) usually feel the fetus move sooner than mothers who are pregnant for the first time (primigravida). The fetus begins to move before the end of the first trimester, but these movements by the relatively small fetus are too slight to be detected by the mother.

8. **D** Placental insufficiency, caused by placental defects (e.g., infarction or nonfunctional areas of the placenta) that reduce the area for passing nutrients to the embryo, produces the placental dysfunction syndrome. Impaired uterine blood flow, caused by severe hypotension and renal disease, can result in a poor passage of nutrients to the embryo. Severe maternal malnutrition resulting from a restricted diet of poor quality may cause low birth weight, especially in teenage mothers. Fetuses of mothers who smoke heavily usually weigh less than fetuses of nonsmokers. Prematurity is a common cause of low birth weight, but full-term fetuses cannot be premature.

9. **C** Withdrawal of samples of amniotic fluid (amniocentesis) is a major tool in assessing the degree of erythroblastosis fetalis (also called hemolytic disease of the fetus). This condition results from destruction of red blood cells by maternal antibodies. Some severely ill fetuses can be saved by giving them intrauterine blood transfusions. Amniotic fluid is also commonly studied to detect chromosomal abnormalities.

10. **A** Ultrasonographic crown-rump measurements are predictive of fetal age with an accuracy of ± 1 to 2 days. The other measurements are also useful for estimating fetal age and size but are less reliable individually. Assessment of fetal age is enhanced when the crown-rump measurements are combined with one or more of these fetal measurements.

Answers and Explanations *Continued*

11. **C** The early development of the external genitalia in both sexes is similar. From the ninth week, the external genitalia passes through an undifferentiated (indifferent) stage, but by the 12th week, distinguishing sexual characteristics are established and a male fetus can easily be differentiated from a female.

12. **A** Ossification begins in the long bones by the eighth week of embryonic development. By the end of the 12th week, primary ossification centers are present in the fetal skeleton, especially in the skull and long bones. Ossification is intense between 13 and 16 weeks, and by the beginning of the 16th week the bones are clearly visible on sonograms taken of the mother's abdomen.

13. **C** Spontaneous fetal movements, known as quickening, are commonly felt by the mother between 17 and 20 weeks. Prior to this period, growth of the fetus is rapid, and by the end of 20 weeks the fetus has a crown-rump length of about 190 mm. The skin of the fetus is covered with vernix caseosa, and hair is present on the head, as well as on the surface of the body. Fetal movement is an important physiologic activity for normal intrauterine development. It also indicates that the fetus is alive. Spontaneous fetal movements can be observed using sonography.

14. **D** The volume of amniotic fluid increases slowly during pregnancy, reaching a peak volume of 1000 ml between 36 and 37 weeks. In about 4% of all pregnancies, the volume of amniotic fluid is markedly reduced, leading to a condition known as oligohydramnios. Sonography is used for diagnosing oligohydramnios because of possible clinical complications. Amniotic fluid is swallowed by the fetus, about 400 ml/day near term. In esophageal atresia, the fetus is unable to swallow amniotic fluid, which accumulates because it cannot pass on to the stomach and intestines for absorption. An increase in the volume of amniotic fluid (>2000 ml) is called polyhydramnios. Oligohydramnios may cause prematurity, fetal compression, and fetal anomalies, such as the amniotic band disruption complex.

15. **B** By 18 weeks, the fetus has a crown-rump length of 160 mm and its smooth skin is covered with vernix caseosa; at 12 weeks the CR length is 120 mm and at 22 weeks it is 210 mm. At this stage of development, the fetus is not viable if born prematurely because its respiratory system is immature for gas exchanges. The presence of fingernails and toenails and open eyes are characteristics of a fetus that is at least 24 weeks old and viable.

16. **D** Lanugo hair is usually absent in an infant with the postmaturity syndrome. Such infants are thin and have a dry parchment skin but are often overweight. At birth, vernix caseosa is decreased or absent, and lanugo hair is lacking. The fingernails are long, and the infants show signs of increased alertness. Prolongation of pregnancy for 3 or more weeks beyond the expected date of confinement occurs in 5 to 6% of women. Some infants in prolonged pregnancies develop the postmaturity syndrome.

■ FIVE-CHOICE ASSOCIATION QUESTIONS

Directions: Each group of questions below consists of a numbered list of descriptive words or phrases accompanied by a diagram with certain parts indicated by letters or by a list of lettered headings. For each numbered word or phrase, **select the lettered part or heading** that matches it correctly and then insert the letter in the space to the right of the appropriate number. Sometimes more than one numbered word or phrase may be correctly matched to the same lettered part or heading.

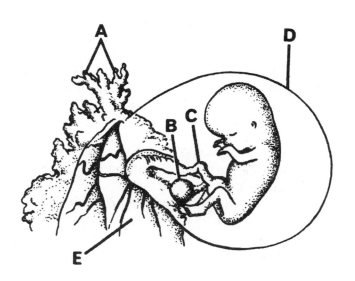

1. _____ Amniotic sac
2. _____ Contains umbilical blood vessels
3. _____ Wall of chorionic sac
4. _____ A vestigial structure
5. _____ Chorionic villi
6. _____ Ensheathed by the amnion

A. 8 to 12 weeks
B. 13 to 16 weeks
C. 17 to 20 weeks
D. 21 to 25 weeks
E. 26 to 29 weeks

7. _____ Skin wrinkled and pink to red
8. _____ Quickening usually occurs
9. _____ Skeleton first shows clearly on x-ray films and sonograms
10. _____ Sex becomes distinguishable externally
11. _____ Eyebrows, head hair, and lanugo hair first visible
12. _____ Head constitutes half the fetus
13. _____ Fetus has good chance of surviving if born prematurely
14. _____ Brown fat begins to form
15. _____ Stage of initial activity of fetus

■ ANSWERS AND EXPLANATIONS

1. **D** The amniotic sac contains amniotic fluid, which permits free movement of the fetus and symmetric external growth. The fluid also cushions the fetus against jolts the mother may receive and helps to control the fetus's body temperature.

2. **C** The umbilical cord contains the umbilical vessels, normally two arteries and one vein. The vein carries nutrients and oxygenated blood to the fetus, and the arteries carry poorly oxygenated blood and waste products to the placenta, where

Answers and Explanations *Continued*

the carbon dioxide and waste substances are transferred to the maternal blood for disposal.

3. **E** The chorionic sac at this stage normally is embedded in the endometrium and contains the embryo in its amniotic sac. Chorionic villi cover most of the outer wall of the sac at this stage. Some villi have degenerated because they were compressed and received insufficient blood supply for survival.

4. **B** The very small remnant of the yolk sac indicated is a vestigial structure, serving no function at this stage. Part of the early yolk sac is incorporated into the embryo during the fourth week as the primordial gut. Within a few weeks, the remnant of the yolk sac indicated degenerates and disappears.

5. **A** The chorionic villi project from the wall of the chorionic sac. These important parts of the placenta normally are embedded in the endometrium and bathed in maternal blood. It is through the villi that the exchange of nutrients between mother and fetus takes place.

6. **C** The umbilical cord has an external investment or covering of amnion. As the amniotic sac enlarges, the amnion gradually forms the outer covering of the cord.

7. **D** During the 21- to 25-week period, the skin usually is wrinkled and pink to red because blood in the capillaries has become visible through the thin, transparent skin. During the subsequent 4 weeks, considerable subcutaneous fat forms, smoothing out many of the wrinkles.

8. **C** During the 17- to 20-week period, movements of the fetus usually are felt by the mother for the first time; this event is known as quickening. Although the fetus begins to move several weeks earlier, the movements are usually too slight to be felt by the mother.

9. **B** Toward the end of the 13- to 16-week period, the skeleton clearly shows on x-ray films. Roentgenography (photography by means of x-rays or roentgen rays) may be used to detect multiple births. Care is taken to prevent the fetus from receiving too much radiation because of the possible adverse effects on its germ cells and developing brain. Sonography is usually used now.

10. **A** Sex first becomes distinguishable during the 8- to 12-week period. At 8 weeks, the external genitalia of males and females appear similar. By the end of the ninth week, it may be is possible to differentiate between males and females, but the mature form of the genitalia is not reached until the 12th week.

11. **C** The 17- to 20-week period is important for several reasons. Fetal movements are first felt by the mother; vernix caseosa forms and affords protection for the fetal skin; body hair (lanugo), head hair, and the eyebrows become visible, and brown fat begins to form. This specialized fat is an important site of heat production.

12. **A** At the beginning of the fetal period, the head constitutes about half the length of the fetus. Thereafter, there is a relative slowdown in the growth of the head compared with the rest of the body. The large head in early fetuses results from the rapid development of the brain during the embryonic period.

13. **E** By the 26- to 29-week period, the fetus has a reasonably good chance of surviving if it is born prematurely, but the mortality rate usually is high because of respiratory difficulties. The fetus is able to survive primarily because its respiratory and nervous systems have matured to the stage where rhythmic breathing can occur. Capillary proliferation in the lungs becomes active during this period. Before the 26- to 28-week period, the pul-

Answers and Explanations *Continued*

monary vascular bed is unable to accommodate the entire cardiac output and so gas exchange in the lungs may not be adequate to support life.

14. **C** Brown fat begins to form during the 17- to 20-week period. Heat is produced in this specialized adipose tissue, particularly during the newborn period, by oxidizing fatty acids. Brown fat is found chiefly at the root of the neck, posterior to the sternum, and in the perirenal regions.

15. **A** The stage of initial activity is during the 8- to 12-week period. By the end of 12 weeks, stroking the lips of a fetus causes it to begin sucking, and if the eyelids are stroked, there is a reflex response. These early movements of the fetus are too slight to be felt by the mother. She usually cannot detect fetal movements until the 17- to 20-week period; these movements, called quickening, constitute a positive sign of a living fetus.

■ NOTES

Placenta and Fetal Membranes

7

Objectives

Be able to:

- Construct and label simple drawings showing the following fetal membranes: amnion, chorion, yolk sac, and allantois. Discuss the fate of each of these fetal membranes.
- Describe the development of the placenta, using drawings to show the essential features of placental structure and function.
- Illustrate the placental membrane (placental barrier), and discuss the transfer of materials between fetal and maternal blood streams.
- List the main activities of the placenta, discussing their role in maintaining pregnancy and promoting embryonic development.
- Construct and label simple drawings showing the gross and microscopic structure of the placenta and umbilical cord after birth.
- Illustrate with sketches and discuss the embryologic basis of multiple births, with special emphasis on twinning.

■ FIVE-CHOICE COMPLETION QUESTIONS

Directions: Each of the following statements or questions is followed by five suggested responses or completions. **Select the one best answer** in each case.

1. Primary chorionic villi are recognizable by the end of the _____ week.
   - A. first
   - B. second
   - C. third
   - D. fourth
   - E. fifth

2. The most distinctive characteristic of a primary chorionic villus is its
   - A. outer syncytial layer
   - B. cytotrophoblastic shell
   - C. mesenchymal core
   - D. cytotrophoblastic core
   - E. villous appearance

3. Villi are designated as secondary chorionic villi when they
   - A. contact the decidua basalis
   - B. are covered by syncytiotrophoblast
   - C. develop a mesenchymal core
   - D. have branch villi
   - E. develop capillaries

Five-Choice Completion Questions *Continued*

4. When villi are vascularized, they are best called _____ villi.
   A. branch
   B. stem
   C. tertiary
   D. anchoring
   E. true

5. The most important region of the decidua for nutrition of the embryo is the decidua _____.
   A. vera
   B. capsularis
   C. parietalis
   D. basalis
   E. none of the above

6. Which of the following regions of the decidua degenerates and disappears during the second trimester of pregnancy?
   A. decidua vera
   B. decidua capsularis
   C. decidua parietalis
   D. decidua basalis
   E. none of the above

7. Contents of the intervillous space normally include each of the following substances *except:*
   A. oxygen
   B. carbon dioxide
   C. maternal blood
   D. fetal blood
   E. electrolytes

8. Which of the following materials usually do not cross the placental membrane (barrier)?
   A. free fatty acids
   B. steroid hormones
   C. bacteria
   D. vitamins
   E. drugs

9. The substance exchanged most rapidly and freely between the mother and her embryo is
   A. water
   B. vitamins
   C. antibodies
   D. free fatty acids
   E. minerals

10. The most characteristic feature of the maternal surface of the placenta is its
    A. attachment of the cord
    B. amniotic covering
    C. cotyledons
    D. shreds of decidua
    E. intervillous spaces

11. At which of the following stages of development is division of embryonic material *not* likely to result in normal monozygotic twinning?
    A. two-cell stage
    B. morula
    C. blastocyst
    D. primitive streak
    E. bilaminar embryo

12. An examination of the placenta and fetal membranes of male twins revealed two amnions, two chorions, and fused placentas. Twinning probably resulted from
    A. dispermy
    B. fertilization of two ova
    C. superfecundation
    D. fertilization of one ovum
    E. the effect of gonadotropins

Five-Choice Completion Questions *Continued*

13. With respect to dizygotic twins, which of the following is correct?
    A. Result from the fertilization of two ova by two sperms
    B. Result from the division of the embryoblast into two primordia
    C. Usually begin to develop during the blastocyst stage
    D. Twins usually are identical.
    E. One chorionic sac is present.

14. Oligohydramnios was diagnosed in a near-term pregnant woman. What type of developmental defect might be present in the fetus?
    A. meroanencephaly
    B. renal agenesis
    C. esophageal atresia
    D. hyaline membrane disease
    E. absence of an umbilical artery

15. Fetal infection may result from the placental transfer of which of the following infectious agents?
    A. cytomegalovirus
    B. Rubella virus
    C. *Toxoplasma gondii*
    D. *Treponema pallidum*
    E. all of the above

16. Most drugs administered during pregnancy are transported across the placental membrane by
    A. simple diffusion
    B. facilitated diffusion
    C. active transport
    D. pinocytosis
    E. none of the above

17. Which of the following does *not* cross the placental membrane?
    A. carbon monoxide
    B. thyroxine
    C. antibodies
    D. uric acid
    E. heparin

18. The average length of the umbilical cord is _____ cm.
    A. 30–40
    B. 40–50
    C. 50–60
    D. 60–70
    E. 70–80

■ ANSWERS AND EXPLANATIONS

1. **B** The appearance of primary chorionic villi is a distinctive feature of the second week of human development. Commencing on about day 9 and continuing until the fourth week, there is intense growth and differentiation of the chorion.

2. **D** Early in the second week, irregular processes of syncytiotrophoblast form; outgrowths of cytotrophoblast soon extend into these syncytiotrophoblast processes. When these primordial villous structures acquire cores of cytotropho-

Answers and Explanations *Continued*

blast, they are called primary chorionic villi. They represent the first stage in the development of the histological structure of the chorionic villi of the mature placenta.

3. **C** The distinctive histological characteristic of a secondary chorionic villus is its loose core of mesenchyme. This embryonic connective tissue is derived from the extraembryonic somatic mesoderm. This change occurs at the end of the second week or early in the third week of development.

4. **C** The final stage in the elaboration of the histological structure of chorionic villi results in the formation of tertiary villi. These villi form the stem (anchoring) villi of the mature placenta. Sometimes the adjective true is used to describe villi in the final stage of development, but tertiary is the better term and the internationally accepted one. Use of the term true villus implies that there are false villi. The arteriocapillary venous system within the core of each villus develops by the end of the third week, and these vessels become connected with those in the chorion, connecting stalk (future umbilical cord), and embryo. Thus, by the end of the third week, a simple circulatory system is established.

5. **D** The gravid (pregnant) endometrium underlying the conceptus, called the decidua basalis, constitutes the maternal part of the placenta. The placenta is primarily an organ for the interchange of material between the maternal and fetal blood streams (e.g., oxygen, carbon dioxide, and food materials).

6. **B** As the conceptus enlarges, the decidua capsularis bulges into the uterine cavity and becomes greatly attenuated. It eventually fuses with the decidua parietalis, obliterating the uterine cavity. By about 22 weeks, reduced blood supply to the decidua capsularis results in its degeneration and subsequent disappearance. Although the epithelium of the decidua parietalis eventually disappears, its other layers persist.

7. **D** There normally is no intermingling of the fetal and maternal blood streams. There is evidence that some fetal and maternal red blood cells cross the placental membrane. The circulation of maternal blood in the intervillous space is of particular importance in the supply of oxygen, electrolytes, and nutrient substances to the fetus and for the removal of its waste products (e.g., carbon dioxide and urea).

8. **C** Bacteria are not transferred across the placenta. Other microorganisms (e.g., rubella virus, cytomegalovirus, and *Toxoplasma gondii*) do cross the placenta and may cause congenital anomalies. When present in the maternal blood, bacteria may form the origin of an infection that subsequently may rupture into the fetal–placental circulation. Almost all substances are probably able to cross the placenta to some extent. It is the rate and the mechanism of crossing that differ. The old sievelike concept of the placenta has been replaced by a more complex view in which the placenta selectively controls the rates of transfer of a wide variety of materials.

9. **A** Water is readily transferred between the mother and the embryo-fetus and in increasing amounts as pregnancy progresses, but the factors that govern the net transfer of water are multiple and complex. Each solute transferred to the embryo and used liberates water molecules. Also, the oxidation of glucose and other nutrients results in the production of water molecules.

10. **C** The 15 to 30 cotyledons give the maternal surface of the placenta a characteristic cobblestone appearance. They are separated by grooves formerly occupied by the placental septa. Although shreds

Answers and Explanations *Continued*

of the decidua basalis are attached to the surface of the cotyledons, they are clearly identifiable only under the microscope. The attachment of the umbilical cord and the amniotic covering are features of the fetal surface of the placenta.

11. **D** After the end of the second week and establishment of a primitive streak, it is unlikely that separate monozygotic twins can develop. If partitioning of the embryonic disc during the second week is incomplete, conjoined twins result. Studies of the chorions, amnions, and placentas of monozygotic twins indicate that most partitioning of embryonic formative material occurs during the blastocyst stage, between days 4 and 7. Separation of the inner cell mass into two parts results in the formation of two embryonic discs, two primitive streaks, and separate embryos.

12. **B** The presence of two chorionic sacs usually indicates dizygotic (dissimilar or fraternal) twinning. From two thirds to three quarters of all human twins are dizygotic. The placentas and membranes observed could be associated with monozygotic twinning because in 25 to 30 per cent of cases, monozygotic twinning results from separation of the first two or more blastomeres. This results in the formation of two amniotic sacs and two chorionic sacs and separate or fused placentas. Thus, it may be difficult to determine if twins with the kind of membranes described are monozygotic or dizygotic. If they are of opposite sex or have different blood types, they are dizygotic. Like-sex twins, as in this case, may be considered monozygotic when they have the same blood type and strongly resemble each other in such characteristics as hair and eye color, fingerprints, and shape of the external ear.

13. **A** Dizygotic twins result from the fertilization of two ova by two sperms. The twins are genetically different and may be of the same sex or different sexes. Monozygotic twins usually develop from the two embryonic primordia formed as a result of the division of the embryoblast during the blastocyst stage. Monozygotic twins are genetically identical and of the same sex. Dizygotic twins have two amnions and two chorions, but the chorions and placentas may be fused. Each monozygotic twin has its own amniotic sac, but they share a common chorionic sac and placenta.

14. **B** Oligohydramnios, or a low volume of amniotic fluid, results in most cases from placental insufficiency, which results in reduced placental blood flow. Renal agenesis is the fetal defect usually associated with this condition because of the lack of fetal urine production. Urine makes a major contribution to the volume of amniotic fluid. The most common cause of oligohydramnios is preterm rupture of the amniochorionic membrane. Meroanencephaly and esophageal atresia are associated with polyhydramnios, or high volumes of amniotic fluid.

15. **E** Cytomegalovirus, rubella virus, and the microorganisms that cause syphillis (*Treponema pallidum*) and toxoplasmosis (*Toxoplasma gondii*) all cross the placenta and may infect the fetus. In some cases, congenital anomalies or death may occur, depending on the infectious agent and the stage of pregnancy.

16. **A** Most drugs are transported across the placental membrane from the mother to the embryo by simple diffusion. The placental transfer of a drug depends on its molecular weight, degree of ionization, and lipid solubility. Some drugs can affect the development of the embryo, leading to major congenital anomalies. Because of the potential risk of damaging the embryo, physicians must weigh the risk against the benefits when prescribing drugs to pregnant women.

Answers and Explanations *Continued*

17. **E** Heparin, an anticoagulant, is not transferred across the placental membrane. Oxygen, carbon dioxide, and carbon monoxide cross the placental membrane by simple diffusion. Thyroxine is essential for the development of the fetus and freely crosses the placental membrane. The nitrogenous waste products urea and uric acid readily cross the placental membrane by simple diffusion and are eventually excreted by the mother.

18. **C** The average length of the umbilical cord is about 55 cm, with a range from 30 to 90 cm. The umbilical cord normally contains two arteries and one vein which transport gases, nutrients, and metabolic waste products between the mother and fetus. Doppler ultrasonography is used for assessing blood flow in the umbilical cord. Fetal complications may follow when the cord is very long or too short. For example, an excessively long cord may prolapse and the blood vessels become compressed, which leads to death of the fetus. A long cord may also become tightly coiled around the limbs or the neck, resulting in strangulation of the fetus. During delivery, a very short cord may result in premature separation of the placenta from its attachment to the endometrium.

■ FIVE-CHOICE ASSOCIATION QUESTIONS

Directions: Each group of questions below consists of a numbered list of descriptive words or phrases accompanied by a diagram with certain parts indicated by letters or by a list of lettered headings. For each numbered word or phrase, **select the lettered part or heading** that matches it correctly and then insert the letter in the space to the right of the appropriate number. Sometimes more than one numbered word or phrase may be correctly matched to the same lettered part or heading.

1. _____ Decidua capsularis
2. _____ Ensheaths the umbilical cord
3. _____ Smooth chorion
4. _____ Decidua parietalis
5. _____ Fuses with the decidua parietalis
6. _____ Maternal part of the placenta

A. Separate placentas and membranes
B. Fibrinoid material
C. Amniochorionic membrane
D. Monochorionic placenta
E. Syncytial knot

7. _____ Occurs only in monozygotic twins
8. _____ Nuclear aggregation
9. _____ Unusual in monozygotic twins
10. _____ Stains intensely with eosin
11. _____ Extends into cervical canal during labor
12. _____ Forms on the surfaces of chorionic villi

Five-Choice Association Questions *Continued*

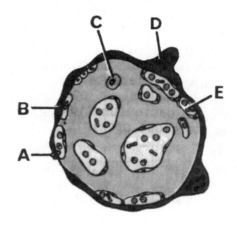

13. _____ Fetal capillary
14. _____ Hofbauer cell
15. _____ Placental membrane
16. _____ Fetal blood
17. _____ Syncytial knot
18. _____ Fibrinoid material

A. Anchoring villi
B. Cytotrophoblast
C. Amnion
D. Battledore placenta
E. Cotyledons

19. _____ Fetal surface of the placenta
20. _____ Largely disappears by birth
21. _____ Features of the maternal surface of the placenta
22. _____ Marginal attachment of the cord
23. _____ Forms part of the early placental membrane
24. _____ Places of attachment to the decidua basalis

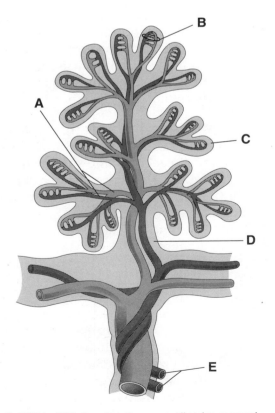

25. _____ Branch villus
26. _____ Fetal capillaries
27. _____ Syncytiotrophoblast
28. _____ Umbilical arteries
29. _____ Arteriocapillary venous network

■ ANSWERS AND EXPLANATIONS

1. **B** The decidua capsularis is the part of the decidua (gravid endometrium) that encapsulates the luminal surface of the implanted conceptus. At the stage shown, it is fused with the smooth chorion. Together the amnion and chorion form the amniochorionic membrane.

2. **D** As the amniotic sac enlarges, it obliterates the chorionic cavity and ensheaths the umbilical cord. The amnion becomes the epithelial covering of the cord.

3. **C** The chorion laeve or smooth chorion is continuous with the chorionic plate (roof) of the placenta. From the third to the eighth week, the region of the chorionic sac indicated is covered by villi. The villi degenerate as the amniotic sac enlarges and presses the chorion against the decidua capsularis. This reduces the blood supply to the villi and results in their degeneration.

4. **A** The decidua parietalis refers to the endometrium lining parts of the uterus not directly involved with the conceptus (i.e., endometrium not designated as decidua capsularis or decidua basalis).

5. **B** The decidua capsularis enlarges with the growing conceptus and bulges into the uterine cavity. The decidua capsularis eventually fuses with the decidua parietalis, thus obliterating the uterine cavity. By about 22 weeks, reduced blood supply to the attenuated decidua capsularis causes it to degenerate and gradually disappear.

6. **E** The decidua basalis forms the maternal part of the placenta. The fetal part is formed by the villous chorion (chorion frondosum). Together they form a unique fetomaternal organ, the placenta, the basic function of which is to bring the maternal and fetal circulations into proximity to permit effective exchange of materials.

7. **D** A monochorionic twin placenta, associated with twins in separate amniotic sacs, occurs only with monozygotic twins; thus, this type of placenta is diagnostic of monozygotic twinning. The twins often have a common fetal-placental circulation that can be demonstrated by injecting colored latex into the vessels of one of the umbilical cords. The latex soon appears in the vessels on the other twin's side of the placenta. This placental condition may produce circulatory imbalance, resulting in diminished blood supply to one of the twins, the so-called transfusion syndrome. With a marked degree of imbalance, considerable differences in the development of the fetuses may occur.

8. **E** At some sites, the syncytiotrophoblast of the placental membrane in mature placentas shows protuberances or sprouts of cytoplasm that contain aggregations of syncytiotrophoblastic nuclei, called syncytial knots. Some knots break off and float in the intervillous space. They may pass into the maternal circulation through the uterine veins and lodge in the capillaries of the lungs. This occurrence is not considered to be of clinical significance because these nuclear masses are believed to degenerate and disappear.

9. **A** Monozygotic twins that develop after separation of the early blastomeres have separate placentas and membranes. Because the early blastocysts are enclosed in the same zona pellucida, they usually implant close together and their chorionic sacs and placentas usually fuse. This arrangement of the placentas and membranes commonly occurs with dizygotic twins. Thus, other criteria must be used to determine what type of twins was born (e.g., comparison of genetic markers such as blood groups or serum factors). A difference in any genetic marker indicates dizygosity. Similarities in several genetic markers do not prove monozygosity because any two children of the same

Answers and Explanations *Continued*

parents might resemble each other in these genetic markers by chance. Many other genetic markers must then be studied before monozygosity is proved or highly probable.

10. **B** Fibrinoid material stains intensely with eosin in hematoxylin–eosin–stained sections of villi. It has been shown to be a mucoprotein-mucopolysaccharide complex. It is present in younger placentas but becomes increasingly abundant in older placentas. It appears at the junction between fetal and maternal tissues, in the chorionic plate (roof of the placenta), and on the surfaces of villi. Fibrinoid material is believed to be important in the prevention of rejection of the placenta and fetus by the mother. These age changes in the material are closely linked with the functional efficiency of the placenta because this amorphous material reduces the surface area of the placental membrane (fetomaternal barrier) available for exchange of materials.

11. **C** The chorion, to which the amnion is fused, extends into the cervical canal during the first stage of labor and helps to dilate the cervix. When the fused layers of amnion and chorion (the amniochorionic membrane) rupture, the amniotic fluid escapes through the cervix and vagina.

12. **B** Fibrinoid is an eosinophilic, homogeneous substance that forms on the surfaces of villi and reduces the area of tissues through which exchange of materials between the maternal and fetal circulations may take place. It consists of fibrin and other unidentified substances.

13. **E** The fetal capillaries, embedded in the stroma of the chorionic villi, are part of an arteriocapillary–venous system that carries the fetal blood. As pregnancy advances, the capillaries increase in size and their walls eventually come into intimate relation with the syncytiotrophoblast. The endothelium of the capillary is separated from the syncytiotrophoblast by only an extremely delicate network of reticular fibers.

14. **C** Hofbauer cells are large cells in the mesenchymal core of chorionic villi. The vacuoles in these cells contain mucopolysaccharides, mucoproteins, and lipids. Although the complete role of these cells is not understood, it is believed that they are macrophages.

15. **A** The placental membrane (barrier) may be defined as the fetal tissues that are interposed between the fetal and placental circulations. The structure and thickness of the membrane vary at different stages of pregnancy. The placental membrane becomes extremely thin as pregnancy advances, and increases in permeability. The thickness of the membrane is also affected by the extent of distention of capillaries in the villus.

16. **E** Poorly deoxygenated blood passes from the fetus in the umbilical arteries. These arteries divide into a number of radially disposed vessels as the cord attaches to the placenta. The arterial branches pass into the chorionic villi and form an extensive arteriocapillary–venous system.

17. **D** Syncytial knots consist of aggregations of nuclei in protuberances of cytoplasm of the syncytiotrophoblast. They form at intervals along a villus; occasionally they break off and enter the maternal circulation. Apparently these nuclear aggregations have a short life in the maternal blood.

18. **B** Fibrinoid material develops as a homogeneous layer at various places on the maternal aspect of the villi. Because it is at the fetomaternal junction of tissues, fibrinoid is believed to be important in preventing rejection of the fetus by the mother. Composed of fibrin and other unidentified substances, fibrinoid decreases

Answers and Explanations *Continued*

the permeability of the placental membrane for exchange of material between the fetal and maternal blood streams.

19. **C** The amnion adheres to the smooth fetal surface of the placenta and is continuous with the epithelial membrane covering the umbilical cord. The umbilical vessels radiate over the fetal surface of the placenta deep to the amnion.

20. **B** The cytotrophoblast layer (Langhans' layer) begins to retrogress and disappear at about 20 weeks. Some cells of this layer, however, persist until full term.

21. **E** Cotyledons are characteristic features of the maternal surface of the placenta. The placental septa divide the maternal surface into 15 to 30 of these areas, which gives the expelled placenta a cobblestone appearance. During examination of the placenta after delivery, special attention should be given to determining whether the cotyledons are all present and intact. If they are not all recognizable and complete, placental tissue may still be in the uterus and must be removed.

22. **D** When the umbilical cord and vessels are attached to the margin of the placenta, it is called a battledore placenta because of its resemblance to the bat used in the medieval game of battledore and shuttlecock. This is a common variation of placental form. Battledore placenta (marginal insertion of the cord) has some clinical significance because slight bleeding occasionally occurs. It has also been shown that many patients with battledore placentas have premature labor.

23. **B** The cytotrophoblast consists of large, pale cells with relatively large nuclei. Their cytoplasm contains vacuoles and some glycogen. The placenta synthesizes glycogen early in pregnancy, and its declining ability to perform this activity later in pregnancy may be related to the assumption of this function by the fetal

liver and to the retrogression of the cytotrophoblast.

24. **A** The main means of attachment of the conceptus to the uterus is by anchoring stem villi that pass from the chorionic plate to the decidua basalis. Columns of cytotrophoblast cells extend through the syncytiotrophoblast at the tips of these villi and cover the maternal tissue. Soon cytotrophoblast cells from adjacent villi join to form a cytotrophoblastic shell around the conceptus. This shell is also attached to the decidua basalis.

25. **C** The main stem villi give rise to numerous branch villi that are bathed externally by maternal blood in the intervillous spaces. Exchange of gases, nutrients, and waste products between mother and fetus occurs between maternal blood in the intervillous space and fetal vessels in the branch villi.

26. **A** Fetal capillaries are tiny blood vessels in the branch villi that transport deoxygenated blood and waste products from the fetus and carry oxygenated blood and nutrients to the fetus. Exchange of material occurs between the blood in the fetal capillaries and in the intervillous space.

27. **D** The trophoblast gives rise to two layers: an inner cellular layer, the cytotrophoblast, and an outer multinucleated cytoplasmic mass, the syncytiotrophoblast. Cells from the cytotrophoblast proliferate rapidly, migrate into the syncytiotrophoblast, and lose their cell membrane. In implantation, the highly invasive syncytiotrophoblast invades the endometrial stroma and by the end of the second week the blastocyst is fully implanted in the endometrium. At this time, the syncytiotrophoblast begins to produce human chorionic gonadotrophin (hCG), which enters the maternal blood and forms the basis for early pregnancy testing.

28. **E** There are normally two umbilical arteries and one umbilical vein in the um-

Answers, Notes, and Explanations *Continued*

bilical cord. The presence of only one umbilical artery may be associated with congenital anomalies in the fetus, often involving the heart and blood vessels. The umbilical arteries transport poorly oxygenated blood and waste products from the fetus to the placenta.

29. **B** An extensive arteriocapillary venous network is formed within the numerous villi from branches of the umbilical arteries and veins. Only the thin placental membrane separates fetal blood in the arteriocapillary venous plexus from the maternal blood in the intervillous space.

■ NOTES

■ NOTES

Birth Defects 8

Objectives

Be able to:

- Discuss congenital anomalies with special reference to the critical periods of development.
- Define the terms teratology and teratogens.
- Discuss the causes of congenital anomalies under each of the following headings, giving examples of their characteristic anomalous patterns:

    Genetic Factors: Changes in chromosome number (aneuploidy and polyploidy), structural abnormalities (translocation and deletion), and gene mutation

    Environmental Factors: Irradiation, infections, and drugs

    Genetic and Environmental Factors: Multifactorial inheritance

---

■ FIVE-CHOICE COMPLETION QUESTIONS

Directions: Directions: Each of the following statements or questions is followed by five suggested responses or completions. **Select the one best answer** in each case.

1. Major congenital anomalies are present in about _____% of neonates.
    A. 0.5
    B. 3.0
    C. 6.0
    D. 10
    E. 15

2. What percentage of deaths in the neonatal period may be attributed to major congenital anomalies?
    A. 2
    B. 5
    C. 15
    D. 20
    E. 25

3. Most major congenital anomalies result from
    A. numerical chromosomal abnormalities
    B. structural chromosomal abnormalities
    C. mutant genes
    D. infectious agents
    E. none of the above

Five-Choice Completion Questions *Continued*

4. The infectious agent most likely to cause a triad of congenital anomalies consisting of heart defects, cataracts, and deafness is
   A. *Toxoplasma gondii*
   B. varicella (chickenpox)
   C. herpes zoster virus
   D. rubella virus
   E. cytomegalovirus

5. Each of the following microorganisms is known to cause major congenital anomalies *except:*
   A. *Treponema pallidum*
   B. cytomegalovirus
   C. varicella
   D. *Toxoplasma gondii*
   E. rubella virus

6. The frequency, severity, and type of abnormalities produced by the rubella virus usually depend on the
   A. number of previous infections
   B. mother's age
   C. severity of the infection
   D. time of maternal infection
   E. sex and age of the embryo

7. Sex chromatin studies indicate that the frequency of sex chromatin–positive males in the general population is about 1:500. Chromosomal studies reveal that the most common chromosome complement (karyotype) in these males is
   A. 48,XXXY
   B. 47,XXY
   C. 48,XXYY
   D. 49,XXXYY
   E. 49,XXXXY

8. Late maternal age and nondisjunction of chromosomes during gametogenesis often are related. In which of the following syndromes is late maternal age believed to be a major factor?
   A. cri du chat syndrome
   B. Turner syndrome
   C. Klinefelter syndrome
   D. Edward syndrome
   E. Down syndrome

9. Congenital anomalies that result from chromosomal breakage are likely to occur in infants born to mothers who received or used
   A. lysergic acid (LSD)
   B. marijuana
   C. heroin
   D. radiation
   E. none of the above

10. Certain chemical agents exhibit varying degrees of teratogenicity when administered during the embryonic period. Which of the following substances is most likely to cause congenital anomalies in human embryos?
    A. cortisone
    B. aminopterin
    C. potassium iodide
    D. lysergic acid
    E. aspirin

Five-Choice Completion Questions *Continued*

11. Infants with microcephaly are grossly retarded because brain development is rudimentary. The cause of this condition often is uncertain. Known causes of microcephaly include each of the following *except:*

    A. rubella virus
    B. cytomegalovirus
    C. *Toxoplasma gondii*
    D. therapeutic radiation
    E. thalidomide

12. Environmental causes of human congenital anomalies may be prevented, to some extent, with proper counseling. Each of the following would be good advice to give a woman who has just missed a menstrual period and may be pregnant *except:*

    A. take only those drugs that have been prescribed by your doctor.
    B. avoid exposure to large amounts of radiation.
    C. obtain a vaccination for protection against rubella infection.
    D. stay away from people who have infectious diseases.
    E. eat a good-quality diet and do not smoke.

13. Growth deficiency, microcephaly, mental retardation, deafness, and chorioretinitis were observed in an infant during routine examination. Radiologic examination of the skull revealed signs of cerebral calcification. The child's mother said that she had some kind of a viral infection during late pregnancy. Which of the following is involved?

    A. herpes simplex virus
    B. varicella virus
    C. cytomegalovirus
    D. human immunodeficiency virus
    E. rubella virus

14. Which of the following drugs does not cross the placental membrane?

    A. heparin
    B. phenytoin
    C. retinoic acid
    D. insulin
    E. tetracycline

15. A 30-year-old woman gave birth to an infant with mental retardation and other anomalies, which included growth deficiency, microcephaly, short palpebral fissures, maxillary hypoplasia, and a thin upper lip. During her pregnancy, she drank both alcoholic beverages and coffee regularly and smoked a pack of cigarettes daily. Which of the following is probably responsible for the child's condition?

    A. mother's age
    B. alcohol ingestion
    C. cigarette smoking
    D. coffee
    E. genetic factors

16. Infants of mothers who smoke cigarettes heavily during pregnancy are most likely to have

    A. limb anomalies
    B. low birth weight
    C. abnormal external genitalia
    D. facial anomalies
    E. spina bifida

Five-Choice Completion Questions *Continued*

17. Which of the following teratogens is usually associated with tooth defects, such as discoloration of the teeth and hypoplasia of the enamel?
    A. cocaine
    B. thalidomide
    C. alcohol
    D. tetracyclines
    E. methotrexate

18. A pregnant woman ingested an androgenic substance throughout the first trimester. Exposure of the developing fetus to excessive androgens may lead to
    A. labioscrotal fusion
    B. mental retardation
    C. intrauterine growth retardation
    D. cerebral calcification
    E. eye anomalies

19. Congenital heart defect is often associated with each of the following teratogens *except:*
    A. isotretinoin
    B. alcohol
    C. tetracyclines
    D. valproic acid
    E. lithium

20. Which of the following drugs/chemicals is (are) recognized as human teratogens?
    A. warfarin (coumadin)
    B. retinoic acid
    C. phenytoin
    D. tetracycline
    E. all of the above

■ ANSWERS AND EXPLANATIONS

1. **B** It is difficult to obtain an accurate estimate of the incidence of congenital anomalies, but it is generally accepted that 2.7 to 3.0% have a medically significant (i.e., major) congenital defect. If one includes minor abnormalities, the incidence is about 5%. Not all defects are recognized at birth; indeed, if one includes all medically significant anomalies that are recognized by the end of the first year, the incidence increases to more than 6%. This emphasizes that less than half of all major anomalies are detected at birth.

2. **D** About 20% of deaths in the neonatal period can be attributed to the presence of congenital defects (e.g., cardiac anomalies and defects of the central nervous system). More deaths occur in the first month of life than in the remaining months of the first year. Many abnormal fetuses can survive before birth but are unable to adjust to the profound changes associated with the onset of extrauterine life. Failure of the normal changes to occur in the circulatory system results in two of the most common congenital abnormalities of the heart and great vessels (patent foramen ovale and patent ductus arteriosus). In many cases, these abnormalities can be corrected by surgical techniques.

3. **E** Most congenital anomalies result from unknown causes. Probably most of them are caused by an interaction of genetic and environmental factors (multifactorial inheritance). About 25% of anomalies are caused by genetic factors (choices A, B, and C), and the remaining anomalies are caused by environmental agents, such as the rubella virus and drugs.

Answers and Explanations *Continued*

4. **D** Rubella virus is a potent teratogen if present during early pregnancy. About 20% of mothers infected with rubella virus during the first month of pregnancy give birth to defective infants. This is understandable because the heart, eyes, and internal ears are developing at this time. The risk of anomalies from infections during the second and third trimesters is low, but functional defects of the nervous system (e.g., mental retardation) and the internal ears may result from infections as late as the 25th week.

5. **C** Varicella virus is known to cross the placenta and infect the fetus. No maternal antibodies confer immunity on the fetus as occurs for smallpox. The other microorganisms listed all produce major congenital defects. Rubella virus produces its effects mainly during the embryonic period, whereas the syphilis organism, cytomegalovirus, and the parasite *Toxoplasma gondii* all produce their effects during the fetal period.

6. **D** The timing of the rubella infection is the most important factor. Infections early in pregnancy cause the most serious defects. Thus, the extent of damage to the embryo varies with the timing of the maternal infection. Severe infections of the mother early in pregnancy often result in abortion; milder infections may result in congenital anomalies.

7. **B** Newborn males with this chromosomal abnormality appear normal. By puberty, they develop Klinefelter syndrome: small testes and hyalinization of the seminiferous tubules. Secondary sexual characteristics usually are poorly developed, and many of these males are tall and eunuchoid. Subnormal mentality is common, especially in people with more than three sex chromosomes. The chromosomal error (nondisjunction) that results in Klinefelter syndrome typically occurs during the first meiotic division of maternal oogenesis, but it can occur during paternal spermatogenesis. In males with four X chromosomes, nondisjunction occurs during the first and second meiotic divisions.

8. **E** It is well established that the frequency of Down syndrome increases with maternal age. As far as is known, late paternal age has little effect on nondisjunction. The frequency of this chromosomal error in mothers may be related to the circumstance that the primary oocytes are formed before birth and remain in the first meiotic prophase until just before ovulation. There is no major maternal-age effect in the other syndromes listed.

9. **D** Most structural abnormalities result from chromosomal breaks induced by various environmental agents, especially large doses of radiation. Certain viruses have also been shown to cause fragmentation of chromosomes, but there is no conclusive evidence that these chromosomal aberrations produce congenital defects. Similarly, it is known that LSD and marijuana can cause chromosomal damage, but there is no conclusive evidence to indicate that these drugs are teratogenic. Heroin is not known to cause chromosomal breakage, but it often causes narcotic addiction in neonates.

10. **B** Aminopterin is a potent teratogen, as are other tumor-inhibiting chemicals (e.g., methotrexate). Potassium iodide may cause congenital goiter and the other substances listed may be weak teratogens, but there is not enough evidence to warrant inclusion of them in a list of known teratogens.

11. **E** Thalidomide is a highly potent teratogen, producing limb defects, deafness, and anomalies of the cardiovascular and digestive systems, but it does not produce microcephaly, mental retardation, or other defects of the central nervous sys-

Answers and Explanations *Continued*

tem. All the other environmental agents listed are known to cause microcephaly.

12. **C** It would be poor advice to recommend vaccination for any disease during early pregnancy. Although there is no conclusive information about the teratogenic potential of live attenuated rubella virus, it is contraindicated. Women should be immunized with live attenuated virus only when pregnancy is not planned during the next 2 months.

13. **C** These are characteristic features of congenital cytomegalovirus infection, which is the most common viral infection of the human fetus. Other findings may include blindness and hepatosplenomegaly, as well as audiologic and neurobehavioral disturbances.

14. **A** Heparin does not cross the placental membrane. It is the drug of choice for pregnant women who require anticoagulant therapy. Molecular weight, degree of ionization, and lipid solubility are some factors that determine the placental transfer of a drug or chemical. The consumption of drugs during pregnancy is surprisingly high, and almost all drugs taken by the mother reach the embryo or fetus. Although relatively few drugs are proven human teratogens, possible adverse effects on the unborn child should be taken into consideration when drugs are used during pregnancy.

15. **B** The findings in the infant are characteristic features of the fetal alcohol syndrome, now considered to be the most common cause of mental retardation in infancy. Although cigarette smoking is known to cause intrauterine growth retardation, like caffeine, there is no evidence that it is teratogenic in humans. Genetic factors are unlikely to be involved, and this case may require follow-up studies for appropriate counseling.

16. **B** Maternal cigarette smoking is a well-established cause of intrauterine growth retardation (IUGR). Mothers who smoke 20 or more cigarettes daily may deliver prematurely, and their infants usually weigh less than normal. Maternal smoking is also associated with behavioral disturbances and decreased physical growth in the child. Infants of mothers who stop smoking, especially before 16 weeks of gestation, show an improvement in their birth weights. There is little evidence in support of a strong association between maternal smoking and congenital anomalies. Nicotine, a vasoconstrictor, constricts the uterine blood vessels and reduces the transfer of oxygen and nutrients from the mother to the fetus. This leads to chronic hypoxia and IUGR.

17. **D** The use of tetracyclines during the second and third trimester may cause a yellow to brown discoloration of the teeth and hypoplasia of the enamel (pitted appearance). Tetracyclines readily cross the placental membrane and are deposited in the bones and teeth of the fetus, with the potential to affect their growth. Because calcification of most permanent teeth begins at birth and is complete at about 8 years of age, tetracycline therapy during early childhood should be avoided. Maternal use of cocaine, thalidomide, alcohol, and methotrexate is not usually associated with tooth anomalies.

18. **A** Infants who are 46, XX females may appear masculinized at birth because of in utero exposure to androgens and high doses of progestogens during the first trimester of pregnancy. There is a varying degree of labioscrotal swelling, and the clitoris is enlarged. Mental retardation, IUGR, and eye anomalies are associated with several teratogens, such as alcohol and the rubella virus. Cerebral calcification is usually present in an infant infected in utero with the intracellular parasite *Toxoplasma gondii* or with cytomegalovirus.

Answers and Explanations *Continued*

19. **C** Isotretinoin, alcohol, tetracyclines, valproic acid, and lithium are commonly used during pregnancy. Tetracyclines cause discoloration of the teeth and hypoplasia of the tooth enamel in the newborn when taken by the mother during the second and third trimester of gestation. Congenital anomalies of the heart are more often found in infants exposed in utero to isotretinoin, alcohol, valproic acid, and lithium.

20. **E** All of the substances listed are well documented as teratogens in humans. Their use during pregnancy is contraindicated, and inappropriate administration of these drugs could have legal consequences involving the physician. Usually the benefits of a particular drug are weighed against possible risks. Warfarin causes nasal hypoplasia, stippled epiphyses, eye anomalies, and mental retardation in the newborn. Retinoic acid induces craniofacial anomalies, mental retardation, and cardiovascular anomalies. Phenytoin is associated with IUGR, mental retardation, cleft palate, and pharyngeal hypoplasia. Tetracycline, which affects the fetus, causes stained teeth and hypoplasia of the enamel.

■ FIVE-CHOICE ASSOCIATION QUESTIONS

Directions: Each group of questions below consists of a numbered list of descriptive words or phrases. For each numbered word or phrase, **select the lettered part or heading** that matches it correctly and then insert the letter in the space to the right of the appropriate number. Sometimes more than one numbered word or phrase may be correctly matched to the same letter.

A. 47,XXX
B. 45,XO
C. Trisomy 18
D. Trisomy 21
E. 47,XXY

1. _____ Webbed neck and short stature
2. _____ Mental retardation, low-set ears, and early postnatal death
3. _____ Normal female appearance and usually fertile
4. _____ Small testes and hyalinization of the seminiferous tubules
5. _____ The most common numerical autosomal abnormality
6. _____ Female with sex chromatin–negative nuclei
7. _____ Strong association with late maternal age
8. _____ Mental retardation, simian crease, and heart defect
9. _____ Sterile male with sex chromatin–positive nuclei

A. Cytomegalovirus
B. Androgenic agents
C. Thalidomide
D. *Toxoplasma gondii*
E. Aminopterin

10. _____ Antitumor agent and potent teratogen
11. _____ Intracellular parasite found in cats
12. _____ Potent teratogen that affects limb development
13. _____ May cause masculinization of female fetuses
14. _____ Known to cause meroanencephaly (anencephaly)
15. _____ Mother may contract it by eating poorly cooked meat

■ ANSWERS AND EXPLANATIONS

1. **B** Webbed neck and short stature are associated with females with Turner syndrome (ovarian dysgenesis). These females have 44 autosomes and only 1 X chromosome. In the newborn period, these infants usually exhibit marked edema of the feet and webbing of the neck. The ovaries commonly consist of only connective tissue streaks. This condition is not recognized in many of these girls until they reach puberty (12 to 15 years), at which time they seek medical advice about primary amenorrhea (failure of menstruation to begin) and the lack of secondary sex development.

2. **C** Infants with trisomy 18 have multiple major anomalies. Like those with the less common trisomy 13 syndrome, these infants have a severe mental defect and die during early infancy. Trisomy 18 is more severe than Down syndrome, and an excess of females are affected (about 78%).

3. **A** Most females with the triple X chromosome abnormality appear normal and are fertile. These women have two sex chromatin masses in their cells because of the presence of the extra X chromosome. Some triple X females have borne children, all of whom are normal and have normal karyotypes. Most females with four or more X chromosomes are also physically normal but severely retarded.

4. **E** XXY males appear normal at birth. Small testes and hyalinization of the seminiferous tubules are the constant characteristics of postpubertal XXY males with Klinefelter syndrome. The secondary sexual characteristics usually are poorly developed, and many of these males are tall and eunuchoid. Subnormal mentality is common.

5. **D** Trisomy 21 is the most common type of numerical autosomal abnormality, occurring about once in 600 neonates. The cause of the chromosomal abnormality (trisomy of chromosome 21) is nondisjunction during oogenesis, usually in older mothers. About 4 per cent of people with Down syndrome have the extra 21 chromosome attached to another chromosome (usually number 14).

6. **B** Females with Turner syndrome (45,XO) were among the first cases studied when accurate chromosomal analyses became possible in 1958. Sex chromatin studies had shown a few years earlier that these females had chromatin-negative nuclei. Some females with stigmata of Turner syndrome are chromatin positive because they are mosaics (i.e., they have a 45,X cell line and a normal 46,XX cell line).

7. **D** Infants with Down syndrome typically are born to older mothers. The mean maternal age is about 35 years compared with 28 in a control population. The older name for this condition is mongolism, coined because of the somewhat slanting look of the eyes. It is an inappropriate name and should not be used.

8. **D** Infants with Down syndrome are mentally retarded (I.Q. commonly is in the 25 to 50 range) and have a heart defect. The single transverse crease (simian crease) in place of the usual creases is found in about 50% of people with the syndrome. It is also found in people with other chromosomal abnormalities and in about 1% of apparently normal people. The presence of a simian crease does not necessarily indicate a chromosomal abnormality and Down syndrome, but it is a useful criterion when associated with other typical characteristics (hypotonia, epicanthal folds, furrowed and protruding tongue).

9. **E** Males with sex chromatin–positive nuclei have Klinefelter syndrome or a related condition. Newborn males appear normal, but the testes remain abnormally small as puberty approaches owing to hy-

Answers and Explanations *Continued*

alinization of the seminiferous tubules. Consequently, they are sterile. Secondary sexual characteristics develop poorly, and gynecomastia (enlargement of the breasts) may occur. These men typically are tall and eunuchoid and commonly have a subnormal mentality.

10. **E**   Aminopterin, an antitumor agent, is also a potent human teratogen. Methotrexate, a derivative of aminopterin, is also teratogenic. These agents produce a wide range of severe skeletal defects and defects of the central nervous system. Aminopterin may produce meroanencephaly (anencephaly), intrauterine growth retardation, and many other abnormalities.

11. **D**   *Toxoplasma gondii* is an intracellular parasite. It infects many birds and mammals, in addition to some humans. Toxoplasmosis, the disease caused by this microorganism, can be contracted from eating raw meat or through contact with infected animals. The parasite affects the fetus during the second and third trimesters, producing microcephaly, microphthalmia, hydrocephaly, and chorioretinitis.

12. **C**   Thalidomide has been shown to produce severe anomalies in the embryo if taken by the mother during the first tri-

mester. As little as 200 mg of this sedative and antinauseant may cause limb defects, cardiac defects, and ear anomalies.

13. **B**   Androgenic agents and certain progestins administered to prevent abortion may cause masculinization of female fetuses. The substances known to cause these anomalies are ethisterone and norethisterone. All substances with known androgenic properties may cause masculinization if administered during the first trimester of pregnancy.

14. **E**   Aminopterin, an antitumor agent and teratogen, is known to cause meroanencephaly (partial absence of the brain) if administered during the early period of brain development (third to fourth week after fertilization).

15. **D**   A mother may become infected with the parasite *Toxoplasma gondii* by eating raw or poorly cooked meat that contains the microorganism. She may contract toxoplasmosis from infected birds, animals, or people. If the parasite crosses the placental membrane, it causes maldevelopment during the fetal period. It causes microcephaly, microphthalmia, hydrocephaly, and chorioretinitis. There is no proof that the parasite affects development during organogenesis (i.e., during the embryonic period).

Body Cavities, Mesenteries, and Diaphragm

9

Objectives

Be able to:

- Describe, with the aid of diagrams, the development of the intraembryonic coelom and the changes resulting in it from longitudinal and transverse folding of the embryo during the fourth week.
- Give an account of the subdivision or partitioning of the body cavities into (1) the pericardial cavity, (2) the pleural cavities, and (3) the peritoneal cavity.
- Explain, with the aid of diagrams, the formation of the dorsal and ventral mesenteries.
- Construct and label diagrams showing the development of the diaphragm. Discuss its four components, positional changes, and innervation.
- Explain the embryologic basis of congenital diaphragmatic hernia. Discuss the possible effects of this defect on the initiation of respiration at birth.

■ FIVE-CHOICE COMPLETION QUESTIONS

Directions: Each of the following statements or questions is followed by five suggested responses or completions. **Select the one best answer** in each case.

1. Each of the following structures is involved in the development of the diaphragm *except* the
   A. lateral body wall
   B. pleuroperitoneal membranes
   C. septum transversum
   D. pleuropericardial membranes
   E. esophageal mesentery

2. The intraembryonic coelom (embryonic body cavity) is first recognizable during the _____ week after fertilization.
   A. second
   B. third
   C. fourth
   D. fifth
   E. sixth

Five-Choice Completion Questions *Continued*

3. The first component of the developing diaphragm is recognizable at the end of the _____ week of development.

   A. second
   B. third
   C. fourth

   D. fifth
   E. sixth

4. After folding of the embryo, the dorsal mesentery extends from the

   A. cranial part of the foregut to the caudal region
   B. caudal part of the foregut to the cranial part of the hindgut
   C. caudal part of the esophagus to the cloacal region
   D. cranial part of the esophagus to the cloacal region
   E. stomodeum to the proctodeum

5. Failure of closure of the cranial end of the pericardioperitoneal canal results in communication between the pleural cavity on the affected side and the

   A. peritoneal cavity
   B. pericardial cavity
   C. abdominopelvic cavity

   D. other pleural cavity
   E. pelvic cavity

6. Failure of closure of the caudal end of the pericardioperitoneal canal results in communication between the pleural cavity on the affected side and the

   A. peritoneal cavity
   B. pericardial cavity
   C. abdominopelvic cavity

   D. other pleural cavity
   E. pelvic cavity

7. In a 4-week embryo, the developing diaphragm (represented by the septum transversum) is located at the level of the

   A. superior cervical somites
   B. inferior thoracic somites
   C. superior thoracic somites

   D. superior lumbar somites
   E. inferior lumbar somites

8. Most muscle-forming cells (myoblasts) that give rise to the musculature of the diaphragm are derived from mesenchymal cells that originate in the

   A. septum transversum
   B. cervical somites
   C. thoracic somites

   D. lumbar somites
   E. lateral mesoderm

9. The septum transversum gives rise to _____ of the diaphragm.

   A. small intermediate portions
   B. the right and left crura
   C. the central tendon

   D. posterolateral portions
   E. peripheral portions

Five-Choice Completion Questions *Continued*

10. In the 5-week embryo, the ventral mesentery of the primordial gut disappears, *except* where it is attached to the
   A. primitive pharynx
   B. embryonic part of the yolk stalk
   C. caudal region of the hindgut
   D. caudal region of the foregut
   E. cranial region of the midgut

11. A congenital diaphragmatic hernia (CDH) was diagnosed prenatally by ultrasonography. Which of the following structures was probably involved?
   A. septum transversum
   B. costodiaphragmatic recess
   C. pleuroperitoneal membrane
   D. dorsal mesentery of the esophagus
   E. lateral body wall

12. Each of the following is derived from the intraembryonic coelom *except* the
   A. peritoneal cavity
   B. extraembryonic coelom
   C. right pericardioperitoneal canal
   D. left pericardioperitoneal canal
   E. pericardial cavity

13. The intraembryonic coelom is connected with the extraembryonic coelom until week _____, after which they become separated.
   A. 6
   B. 8
   C. 10
   D. 12
   E. 14

■ ANSWERS AND EXPLANATIONS

1. **D** The pleuropericardial membranes are not involved in the formation of the diaphragm. They form partitions at the cranial ends of the pericardioperitoneal canals and separate the pericardial cavity from the pleural cavities. The other four structures listed are the main components of the developing diaphragm.

2. **B** Intercellular spaces, lined by mesothelium, appear in the lateral mesoderm and cardiogenic mesoderm 18 to 19 days after fertilization. These spaces coalesce to form the intraembryonic coelom, a horseshoe-shaped cavity within the lateral mesoderm and cardiogenic mesoderm in the human embryonic disc.

3. **B** The septum transversum is the first recognizable component of the developing diaphragm. It appears at the end of the third week as a mass of mesoderm cranial to the pericardial coelom. After the head fold occurs during the fourth week, the septum transversum forms a thick mass of mesenchyme between the thoracic and abdominopelvic cavities. Later it becomes extensively invaded by the developing liver and eventually becomes a thin layer (the primordium of the central tendon) between the pericardial cavity and the liver.

4. **C** The dorsal mesentery extends from the caudal part (inferior end) of the esophagus to the cloacal region of the hindgut. In the region of the esophagus, the mesentery is called the mesoesophagus; in the stomach region, it is called the dorsal mesogastrium or greater omentum; and in the region of the colon, it is called mesocolon. The dorsal mesentery

Answers and Explanations *Continued*

of the jejunum and ileum is called the mesentery proper. The dorsal mesentery of the duodenum (dorsal mesoduodenum) disappears completely, except in the region of the pylorus of the stomach.

5. **B** Defective formation or fusion of the pleuropericardial membrane, usually on the left side, is uncommon. When this occurs, there is a defect in the fibrous pericardium, the adult derivative of the pleuropericardial membranes. Part of the left atrium may herniate into the left pleural cavity if there is a defect in the pericardium.

6. **A** Defective formation or fusion of the pleuroperitoneal membrane, usually on the left side, is relatively common (occurs about once in 2200 births). This results in a posterolateral defect in the diaphragm through which abdominal viscera may herniate into the thorax. Congenital diaphragmatic hernia usually constitutes a medical-surgical emergency in the newborn period because of respiratory disorders (pressure on the lungs, causing poor lung expansion and difficult breathing).

7. **A** As the head fold forms, the septum transversum and the pericardial cavity move into a ventral position. When it lies opposite to the upper cervical segments of the spinal cord, nerves from the third, fourth, and fifth segments grow into the septum transversum, forming the phrenic nerves. These nerves are the sole motor nerve supply to the diaphragm and are also sensory to the central part of the diaphragm derived from the septum transversum. In the later weeks of development, the diaphragm descends, so that the dorsal part reaches the level of the first lumbar vertebra by the end of the embryonic period.

8. **B** Most of the musculature of the diaphragm is thought to be derived from mesenchymal cells that originate in the myotome regions of the cervical somites.

When these cells migrate into the septum transversum with the developing phrenic nerves, they differentiate into myoblasts (developing muscle fibers). When the developing diaphragm migrates caudally during subsequent development, the phrenic nerves supplying these muscles follow the diaphragm caudally. Some myoblasts probably differentiate from mesenchymal cells in the septum transversum. Other myoblasts probably arise from mesenchymal cells that migrate from the thoracic somites and enter the diaphragm with the lateral body wall tissues that split off when the pleural cavities enlarge by invading the chest wall.

9. **C** The septum transversum gives rise to the central tendon of the diaphragm. Small intermediate portions of it are derived from the pleuroperitoneal membranes, and the crura develop from the growth of muscle fibers into the dorsal mesentery of the esophagus. The peripheral portions of the diaphragm are derived from lateral body wall tissue that is split off as the lungs and pleural cavities enlarge and burrow into the lateral body walls.

10. **D** The ventral mesentery disappears except where it is attached to the caudal (inferior) part of the foregut. This region gives rise to the terminal portion of the esophagus, the stomach, and the superior part of the duodenum. Caudal to the bile duct, the intestines have no ventral mesentery. When most of the ventral mesentery disappears, the right and left peritoneal cavities become a continuous large peritoneal sac in which the viscera are suspended by the dorsal mesentery.

11. **C** Congenital diaphragmatic hernia usually results from failure of the pleuroperitoneal membrane to fuse with the dorsal mesentery of the esophagus and the septum transversum. Mesoderm of the septum transversum forms the central tendon of the diaphragm. The primordial

Answers and Explanations *Continued*

diaphragm between the thoracic and abdominal cavities is established after fusion of the pleuroperitoneal membranes with the septum transversum and the dorsal mesentery of the esophagus. The inner layer of the body wall contributes muscle fibers to the peripheral parts of the diaphragm. Posterolateral defect of the diaphragm is the most common anomaly of the diaphragm, and it occurs more frequently on the left side. This defect permits herniation of abdominal viscera into the thoracic cavity, which causes compression (hypoplasia) of the lung. The prognosis is poor because of the resulting severe respiratory distress and other complications.

12. **B** The extraembryonic coelom is a large cavity formed within the extraembryonic mesoderm during the second week. It is not derived from the intraembryonic coelom, even though they communicate with each other. The intraembryonic coelom arises during the third week from isolated coelomic spaces in the lateral mesoderm and in the cardiogenic mesoderm. These coelomic spaces coalesce to form a horseshoe-shaped cavity that gives rise to the large peritoneal cavity, the two pericardioperitoneal canals (future pleural cavities), and the pericardial cavity.

13. **C** The peritoneal part of the intraembryonic coelom becomes separated from the extraembryonic coelom in the 10th week. The intraembryonic coelom gives rise to the peritoneal cavity, the pleural cavities, and the pericardial cavity. The distal end of each limb of the horseshoe-shaped intraembryonic coelom opens into the extraembryonic coelom at the lateral edges of the embryonic disc. This communication is important because the midgut herniates through it into the umbilical cord, where the midgut develops into most of the small and large intestine. During the 10th week, as the intestine returns to the abdomen from the umbilical cord, the peritoneal cavity becomes separated from the extraembryonic coelom.

■ FIVE-CHOICE ASSOCIATION QUESTIONS

Directions: Each group of questions below consists of a numbered list of descriptive words or phrases accompanied by a diagram with certain parts indicated by letters or by a list of lettered headings. For each numbered word or phrase, **select the lettered part or heading** that matches it correctly and then insert the letter in the space to the right of the appropriate number. Sometimes more than one numbered word or phrase may be correctly matched to the same lettered part or heading.

1. _____ Disappears caudally
2. _____ Derived from the intraembryonic coelom
3. _____ Ventral mesentery of the stomach
4. _____ Caudal part of the foregut
5. _____ Dorsal mesogastrium

Five-Choice Association Questions *Continued*

A. Costodiaphragmatic recess
B. Cervical myotomes
C. Congenital hiatal hernia
D. Pleuroperitoneal membrane
E. Pericardioperitoneal canal

6. _____ Large esophageal opening
7. _____ Extension of the pleural cavity
8. _____ Posterolateral diaphragmatic defect
9. _____ Diaphragmatic muscles
10. _____ Connects the pericardial and peritoneal cavities
11. _____ Herniation of the abdominal viscera

A. Esophageal mesentery
B. Pleuropericardial membrane
C. Phrenic nerves
D. Crura of the diaphragm
E. Embryonic mediastinum

12. _____ Derived from the third to fifth cervical cord segments
13. _____ Common cardinal vein
14. _____ Muscular origins of the diaphragm
15. _____ Mesenchyme separating the lungs
16. _____ Forms the median portion of the diaphragm

17. _____ Future pleural cavity
18. _____ Primordium of the esophagus
19. _____ Produces mesenchyme
20. _____ Gives rise to the central tendon
21. _____ Located caudal to the heart

22. _____ Pleuroperitoneal membrane
23. _____ Derived from the foregut
24. _____ Esophageal mesentery
25. _____ Future pleural cavity
26. _____ Gives rise to the central tendon

■ ANSWERS AND EXPLANATIONS

1. **A** The ventral mesentery disappears caudal to the superior or first part of the duodenum. Note that the liver is developing between the layers of the ventral mesentery. The ventral mesentery forms during transverse folding of the embryo and gives rise to (1) the lesser omentum, (2) the falciform ligament, and (3) the visceral peritoneum of the liver.

2. **E** The peritoneal cavity is derived from the caudal extension of the horseshoe-

Answers and Explanations *Continued*

shaped intraembryonic coelom that forms early in the fourth week of development. In the illustration, the foregut (developing stomach) is suspended in the peritoneal cavity by the dorsal mesentery (dorsal mesogastrium) and the ventral mesentery (hepatogastric ligament).

3. **A** The ventral mesentery (mesogastrium) of the stomach develops from the septum transversum and extends from this septum to the ventral aspect of the caudal part of the foregut. This part of the foregut gives rise to the stomach and the superior part of the duodenum. After the liver develops, the ventral mesentery attaches the stomach to the liver (hepatogastric ligament) and the first part of the duodenum to the liver (hepatoduodenal ligament).

4. **B** The endoderm of the caudal part of the foregut gives rise to the epithelium and glands of the inferior end of the esophagus, the stomach, and the superior part of the duodenum. The muscular and fibrous elements of these structures are derived from the surrounding splanchnic mesoderm. The superior part of the foregut gives rise to the pharynx and its derivatives, the lower respiratory tract, and the superior part of the esophagus.

5. **D** The dorsal mesentery (mesogastrium) of the stomach suspends the stomach in the peritoneal cavity. The spleen subsequently develops between the two layers of the dorsal mesogastrium. Later, as the result of positional changes and growth, the dorsal mesogastrium hangs over the transverse colon and the small intestines, from which it hangs like an apron; this portion of the dorsal mesentery is called the greater omentum.

6. **C** If the embryonic esophageal hiatus or opening in the diaphragm is excessively large, abdominal viscera may herniate through it into the thorax, producing a congenital hiatal hernia. Another uncom-

mon type of CDH, the esophageal hernia, is believed to be caused by a short esophagus. Because of this anomaly, the superior part of the stomach remains in the thorax and the stomach is constricted where it passes through the esophageal opening.

7. **A** As the pleural cavities enlarge, they extend into the body walls, forming costodiaphragmatic recesses. This excavation process also splits off body wall tissue, which contributes to peripheral portions of the diaphragm and establishes the characteristic dome-shaped configuration of the diaphragm.

8. **D** If the pleuroperitoneal membrane fails to develop or to fuse with other parts of the diaphragm, a posterolateral defect develops, usually on the left side. Associated with this defect is herniation of abdominal viscera into the thorax and compression of the lungs. This type of CDH often results in a medical-surgical emergency because of difficulty in breathing.

9. **B** The diaphragmatic muscles are mainly derived from myoblasts that migrate from the myotome regions of the cervical somites. Other myoblasts are derived from the myotome regions of the thoracic somites, and some myoblasts originate in the body wall tissues.

10. **E** The pericardioperitoneal canals give rise to the adult pleural cavities. Membranes develop at the cranial and caudal ends of these canals that separate the pleural cavities from the pericardial cavity and the peritoneal cavity, respectively. The developing lungs invaginate the medial walls of the pericardioperitoneal cavities. The inner (visceral) and outer (parietal) walls of these canals eventually come close together as the layers of pleura.

Answers and Explanations *Continued*

11. **D** Herniation of abdominal viscera into the thorax occurs through a posterolateral defect in the diaphragm where there is failure of development or fusion of the pleuroperitoneal membrane with other parts of the diaphragm, usually on the left side. Because of the presence of abdominal viscera in the thorax, the lungs often are compressed and may be hypoplastic (incompletely developed).

12. **C** The phrenic nerves are derived from the third, fourth, and fifth cervical segments of the spinal cord. These nerves accompany the myoblasts that grow into the developing diaphragm from the myotome regions of the cervical somites. The diaphragm descends as elongation of the neck, descent of the heart, and expansion of the pericardial and pleural cavities occur. The descent of the diaphragm, after it receives its main nerve supply, explains the rather unusual course of the phrenic nerves.

13. **B** The common cardinal veins, which are the main venous channels entering the heart, are in the pleuropericardial membranes. At first, these membranes appear as small ridges projecting into the pericardioperitoneal canals. They eventually fuse with the mesoderm ventral to the esophagus (primordial mediastinum), closing the connections between the pericardial cavity and the pleural cavities.

14. **D** The crura of the diaphragm (muscular origins of the diaphragm from the superior lumbar vertebrae) develop as muscle fibers within the esophageal mesentery.

15. **E** The mediastinum (median septum) in the embryo consists of a mass of mesenchymal tissue separating the lungs and extending from the sternum to the vertebral column. It forms the median dividing wall of the thoracic cavity and contains all the thoracic viscera and structures except the lungs.

16. **A** The dorsal mesentery of the esophagus (mesoesophagus) forms the median portion of the diaphragm. The pleuroperitoneal membranes fuse with the esophageal mesentery and the septum transversum during the sixth week, forming a partition between the thoracic and abdominal cavities. Completion of the diaphragm occurs during the 9th to 12th weeks as body wall tissue is added to it peripherally.

17. **B** The pericardioperitoneal canals are the future pleural cavities. As the lungs develop, they invaginate (push into) the medial walls of these canals, like fists pushed into the sides of almost empty balloons. These invaginations are so complete that the space between the two walls of the canals (future layers of pleura) is reduced to a narrow gap.

18. **E** The foregut gives rise to the epithelium and glands of the esophagus and stomach. Other regions of the foregut give rise to the pharynx and its derivatives, lower respiratory tract, duodenum as far as the bile duct, liver, pancreas, and biliary apparatus.

19. **C** The somites, derived by division of the paraxial mesoderm, give rise to the mesenchyme that differentiates into most of the axial skeleton and its associated musculature. Mesenchyme is an embryonic connective tissue that gives rise to a wide variety of adult tissues (e.g., fibroblasts, fibrocytes, osteoblasts, osteocytes, chondroblasts, chondrocytes, myoblasts, and muscle fibers).

20. **A** The septum transversum, a thick mass of mesenchyme, gives rise to the central tendon of the diaphragm. It is the first component of the diaphragm to be recognizable (end of third week). It forms the caudal limit of the pericardial cavity after folding of the embryo and separates it from the future peritoneal cavity. During the fourth week, groups of

Answers and Explanations *Continued*

myoblasts (muscle-forming cells) from the cervical somites (three to five) migrate into the cranial part of the septum transversum, carrying their phrenic nerve fibers with them.

21. **A** The septum transversum is located caudal to the heart. Early in the fourth week, it lies cranial to the pericardial coelom and the developing heart. As the brain develops, the head folds ventrally, carrying the septum transversum, developing heart, pericardial coelom, and the oropharyngeal membrane ventral to the foregut.

22. **D** The pleuroperitoneal membranes, produced as the lungs and pleural cavities expand by invading the body walls, form caudal partitions in the pericardioperitoneal canals. These membranes gradually grow medially and fuse during the sixth week with the dorsal mesentery of the esophagus and the septum transversum to form the diaphragm. Failure of one of these membranes to form results in a CDH through which the abdominal viscera can herniate. The defect usually appears in the region of the left kidney.

23. **C** The epithelium and the glands of the esophagus are derived from the foregut. The muscular and fibrous elements of the esophagus are derived from the surrounding splanchnic mesenchyme. The foregut also gives rise to the epithelium and the glands of the lower respiratory tract. Faulty partitioning of the foregut into the esophagus and trachea during the fourth and fifth weeks results in a tracheoesophageal fistula.

24. **E** The esophageal mesentery (dorsal mesentery of the esophagus) is one of the components of the primordial diaphragm. The other components are the septum transversum and the pleuroperitoneal membranes. Later, a fourth component, the body wall, contributes to peripheral regions of the diaphragm. The esophageal mesentery constitutes the median portion of the diaphragm. The crura of the diaphragm develop from muscle fibers that form in the dorsal mesentery of the esophagus.

25. **A** The pericardioperitoneal canals become the pleural cavities. The bronchial buds grow laterally during the fifth week and evaginate the medial walls of the canals. The inner walls of the canals become the visceral pleura and the outer walls become the parietal pleura.

26. **B** The septum transversum gives rise to the central tendon of the diaphragm. It is a thick mass of mesenchyme located caudal to the developing heart. Although initially located opposite the cervical region of the spinal cord, the septum transversum is invaded by myoblasts from the third, fourth, and fifth myotome regions of the cervical somites. Later, the diaphragm descends until its dorsal part lies at the level of the first lumbar vertebra. Thus, the seemingly curious origin and course of the phrenic nerves result from the developmental origin of the septum transversum.

The Pharyngeal (Branchial) Apparatus

10

Objectives

Be able to:

- Explain what is meant by the term pharyngeal (branchial) apparatus.
- List and illustrate the components of the pharyngeal (branchial) arches.
- Construct and label diagrams showing the derivatives of the pharyngeal (branchial) arch cartilages.
- Discuss the formation of the pharyngeal pouches, indicating their adult derivatives.
- Describe the development of the tongue and the thyroid gland.
- Discuss the embryological basis of ectopic thyroid gland, thyroglossal duct cysts, and sinuses.
- Illustrate the development of the face and palate, describing the embryological basis of cleft lip and cleft palate.
- Write brief notes on branchial cysts, sinuses, and fistulas; first arch syndrome; and DiGeorge syndrome.

■ FIVE-CHOICE COMPLETION QUESTIONS

Directions: Each of the following statements or questions is followed by five suggested responses or completions. **Select the one best answer** in each case.

1. The pharyngeal (branchial) apparatus is composed of
   A. pharyngeal grooves
   B. pharyngeal arches
   C. pharyngeal pouches
   D. pharyngeal membranes
   E. all the above

2. The third pharyngeal arch cartilage gives rise to which of the following structures?
   A. stylohyoid ligament
   B. thyroid cartilage
   C. styloid process
   D. sphenomandibular ligament
   E. greater cornu of hyoid bone

3. Which of the following structures is *not* related to the first pharyngeal arch?
   A. malleus
   B. facial nerve
   C. Meckel cartilage
   D. mandibular prominence
   E. maxillary prominence

Five-Choice Completion Questions *Continued*

4. Which of the following structures is *not* derived from the second pharyngeal arch cartilage?
   A. incus
   B. stapes
   C. styloid process
   D. lesser cornu of hyoid bone
   E. superior part of hyoid bone

5. Pharyngeal arches are first recognizable around the middle of the _____ week of development.
   A. third
   B. fourth
   C. fifth
   D. sixth
   E. none of the above

6. The cartilages of the larynx are derived mainly from the cartilages of which of the following pharyngeal arches?
   A. second and third
   B. third and fourth
   C. third, fourth, and fifth
   D. fourth and sixth
   E. fourth and fifth

7. Muscle elements in the second pair of pharyngeal arches give rise to which of the following muscles?
   A. frontalis
   B. platysma
   C. orbicularis oculi
   D. buccinator
   E. all of the above

8. Which of the following cranial nerves supplies muscles derived from the first pair of pharyngeal arches?
   A. vagus
   B. glossopharyngeal
   C. facial
   D. trigeminal
   E. none of the above

9. How many *well-defined* pairs of human pharyngeal pouches develop?
   A. two
   B. three
   C. four
   D. five
   E. six

10. Structures derived from the first pharyngeal pouch include
    A. tympanic antrum
    B. tympanic cavity
    C. tubotympanic recess
    D. pharyngotympanic tube
    E. all of the above

11. The most common congenital anomaly of the head and neck is
    A. cleft palate
    B. bilateral cleft lip
    C. oblique facial cleft
    D. unilateral cleft lip
    E. median cleft lip

12. Which of the following structures is derived from the fourth pair of pharyngeal pouches?
    A. thymic corpuscles
    B. superior parathyroid glands
    C. inferior parathyroid glands
    D. thymus
    E. all of the above

Five-Choice Completion Questions *Continued*

13. A young infant had a small blind pit on the side of the neck along the anterior border of the sternocleidomastoid muscle. Mucus dripped intermittently from its opening. What is the most likely embryological basis of this congenital anomaly of the neck? Persistence of the embryonic opening of the
    A. second pharyngeal pouch
    B. second pouch and groove
    C. third pharyngeal groove
    D. thyroglossal duct
    E. second groove and cervical sinus

14. Cleft lip, with or without cleft palate, occurs about once in 1000 births. Which of the following is considered to be an important causative factor in the production of this anomaly?
    A. riboflavin deficiency
    B. infectious disease
    C. mutant genes
    D. cortisone
    E. irradiation

15. The major portion of the human palate develops from the
    A. lateral palatine processes
    B. median palatine process
    C. intermaxillary segment
    D. medial nasal prominences
    E. frontonasal elevation

16. In DiGeorge syndrome, the development of the thymus is affected. Which of the following is involved?
    A. first pharyngeal pouch
    B. second pharyngeal pouch
    C. third pharyngeal pouch
    D. fourth pharyngeal pouch
    E. none of the above

17. When the palatine processes (palatal shelves) fail to meet and fuse with each other and with the nasal septum, the resulting anomaly is a cleft of the
    A. uvula
    B. primary palate
    C. secondary palate
    D. primary and secondary palates
    E. intermaxillary segment

18. The greater cornu and inferior part of the hyoid bone were absent at birth. Which of the following embryonic structures was affected?
    A. maxillary prominence
    B. mandibular prominence
    C. second pharyngeal arch
    D. third pharyngeal arch
    E. fourth pharyngeal arch

19. Which of the following is correct with reference to the developing face?
    A. Unilateral cleft lip results from failure of the medial nasal prominences to merge with each other.
    B. The nasolacrimal duct develops along the groove between the maxillary and lateral nasal prominences.
    C. The intermaxillary segment of the upper jaw is formed when the maxillary prominences merge with one another.
    D. Cleft lip occurs more frequently in females.
    E. All of the above.

Five-Choice Completion Questions *Continued*

20. With respect to the development of the palate, each of the following is correct *except:*
    A. If both lateral palatine processes fuse with the median palatine process but fail to fuse with the nasal septum and each other, a bilateral cleft of the secondary or posterior palate results.
    B. The palatine processes are derived from the maxillary and merged medial nasal prominences.
    C. Ossification of the palate does not extend posterior to the nasal septum.
    D. Fusion of the palatine processes begins in the sixth week.
    E. The primary palate develops from the intermaxillary segment of the maxilla.

21. The external acoustic meatus develops from the
    A. first pharyngeal groove
    B. second pharyngeal groove
    C. first pharyngeal pouch
    D. second pharyngeal pouch
    E. none of the above

22. Concerning cleft of the upper lip, which of the following is correct?
    A. The incidence is about 1 in 1000 live births.
    B. It occurs more frequently in males than females.
    C. It results from failure of fusion/merging between the maxillary prominence and the merged medial nasal prominences.
    D. It is embryologically distinct from a cleft palate.
    E. All of the above.

23. An infant was diagnosed as having a primary cleft of the palate. This congenital defect is
    A. located anterior to the incisive fossa
    B. caused by failure of the lateral palatine processes to fuse with each other
    C. located posterior to the incisive fossa
    D. more common in males than in females
    E. due to the absence of lateral nasal prominences

Five-Choice Completion Questions *Continued*

24. A 30-year-old woman visited her doctor because of a painless swelling on the right side of her neck. A CT scan revealed a well-defined cystic mass at the angle of the mandible, just anterior to the sternocleidomastoid muscle. The most likely diagnosis is
    A. lateral cervical cyst
    B. thyroglossal duct cyst
    C. dermoid cyst
    D. swollen lymph node
    E. accessory thyroid tissue

■ ANSWERS AND EXPLANATIONS

1. **E**   Pharyngeal (branchial) arches, grooves (clefts), and membranes as well as pharyngeal pouches of the cranial end of the foregut (primordial pharynx) are parts of the human pharyngeal apparatus that develops during the fourth week. This apparatus subsequently is transformed into various structures in the head and neck. For example, the pharyngeal pouches become modified to form structures like the tympanic cavity and the parathyroid and thymus glands.

2. **E**   The cartilages of the third pair of pharyngeal arches give rise to the greater cornua of the hyoid bone and to the inferior part of the body of this bone. The lesser cornua and the superior part of the body of the hyoid bone are derived from the second pharyngeal arch cartilages.

3. **B**   The facial nerve is not a component of the first or mandibular arch; it is the nerve of the second or hyoid arch. The nerve of the first or mandibular arch is the trigeminal nerve (CN V). The malleus is derived from the dorsal end of the first arch cartilage. The mandibular prominence is the larger of the two prominences of the first arch; it forms one side of the mandible. The maxillary prominence of the first arch, smaller than the mandibular prominence, contributes to the maxilla. Meckel cartilage is the name

often given to the first arch cartilage; it gives rise to two middle ear bones (malleus and incus), but the mandible forms by intramembranous bone formation around the Meckel cartilage as it degenerates.

4. **A**   The incus is not derived from the second pharyngeal arch cartilage. It is formed by endochondral ossification of the dorsal end of the first arch cartilage (Meckel cartilage). In addition to the derivatives of the second arch cartilage listed, the stylohyoid ligament is derived from its perichondrium.

5. **B**   The first and second pairs of pharyngeal arches are visible on each side of the future head and neck region by about 24 days. The third pair is recognizable by 26 days, and four pairs are present by the end of the fourth week. The fifth and sixth pairs of arches are rudimentary and are not recognizable externally. As the pharyngeal arches form, the endoderm of the primordial pharynx bulges outward between adjacent arches to form the pharyngeal pouches.

6. **D**   The thyroid, cricoid, arytenoid, corniculate, and cuneiform cartilages are derived mainly from the fused cartilages of the fourth and sixth arch cartilages. The fifth pharyngeal arch is rudimentary and

Answers and Explanations *Continued*

soon degenerates; often it does not develop. The cartilage in the epiglottis develops later than the other cartilages from mesenchyme derived from the hypobranchial eminence, a derivative of the third and fourth pair of pharyngeal arches.

7. **E**   All of these muscles are derived from myoblasts that differentiate from mesenchyme in the second pair of pharyngeal arches. During development, some myoblasts from the second arch migrate into the head, mainly to the facial region, and give rise to the muscles of facial expression. During their extensive migration, the developing muscles take their nerve supply (facial nerve) with them from the second arch.

8. **D**   The fifth cranial nerve (trigeminal nerve) supplies the muscles of mastication and other muscles derived from myoblasts in the first pharyngeal (branchial) arch. Because it supplies pharyngeal muscles, the trigeminal nerve and other arch nerves are classified as branchial nerves. Because mesenchyme from the arches also contributes to the dermis and mucous membranes of the head and neck, these areas are supplied with sensory or branchial afferent fibers in the same nerve. The ophthalmic division of the trigeminal nerve does not supply arch derivatives.

9. **C**   There are four well-defined pairs of pharyngeal pouches. The fifth pair is rudimentary or does not form; if present, they either disappear or are incorporated into the fourth pharyngeal pair of pouches to form the so-called caudal pharyngeal complex.

10. **E**   All of these structures are derived from the first pharyngeal pouch. The pouch expands into an elongate, tubotympanic recess that envelops the middle ear bones (auditory ossicles) derived from the dorsal ends of the first and second arch cartilages. The stalk of the recess gives rise to the lining of the pharyngotympanic tube, and the expanded distal part becomes the lining of the tympanic cavity and antrum of the middle ear.

11. **D**   Cleft lip, with or without cleft palate, occurs about once in 1000 births. Unilateral cleft lip is more common than bilateral cleft lip. Cleft palate, with or without cleft lip, occurs about once in 2500 births. Median cleft lip and oblique facial clefts are uncommon congenital anomalies. Cleft lip and cleft palate are embryologically and etiologically distinct anomalies.

12. **B**   The superior parathyroid glands are derived from the fourth pair of pharyngeal pouches. All the other structures are derived from the third pair of pouches. One would think that the superior parathyroid glands would be derived from the third rather than the fourth pair of pouches. The reason they are not is that the parathyroids from the third pair of pharyngeal pouches are attached to the thymus and descend with it to a more inferior level than the parathyroids derived from the fourth pair of pharyngeal pouches.

13. **E**   The anomaly probably is an external branchial or lateral cervical sinus, resulting from the persistence of the opening into the cervical sinus. During the fifth week, the second pharyngeal (hyoid) arch grows over the third and fourth arches, forming an ectodermal depression known as the cervical sinus. The second pharyngeal groove and the opening into the cervical sinus normally are obliterated as the neck forms. If the opening persists, it usually appears as an external opening on the side of the inferior one third of the neck. If the second pharyngeal pouch and pharyngeal groove persisted (choice **B**), a branchial fistula would form and open on the neck, but these are not so common as branchial si-

Answers and Explanations *Continued*

nuses. Thyroglossal duct sinuses, formed after infection of a thyroglossal duct cyst, usually open in the median plane of the neck anterior to the laryngeal cartilages.

14. **C** Cleft lip in animals appears to have a mixed genetic and environmental causation, but practically nothing is known about environmental factors that may be involved in the production of the anomaly in human embryos. A riboflavin-deficient diet given to pregnant rats produces cleft lip in the fetuses, but it is not known to be a causative factor in humans. Experimental work in mice has consistently shown that cortisone causes cleft palate in a high incidence of fetuses, but it is not known to cause cleft lip in mouse or human embryos. Studies in humans indicate that genetic factors are of more importance in cleft lip, with or without cleft palate, than in cleft palate alone. If the parents are normal and have one child with a cleft lip, the chance that the next child will have a cleft lip is 4 per cent. If one of the parents has cleft lip and they have a child with a cleft lip, the probability that the next child will be affected is 17 per cent. Thus, mutant genes appear to be the most important causative factors.

15. **A** The lateral palatine processes (palatal shelves) of the maxillary prominences of the first pair of pharyngeal arches give rise to the posterior or secondary palate. The primary palate or median palatine process develops from the innermost portion of the intermaxillary segment of the upper jaw. This segment, derived from the merged medial nasal prominences, gives rise to the small premaxillary region of the palate.

16. **C** In DiGeorge syndrome, the thymus and parathyroid glands are absent. Other anomalies are also present. The thymus develops from endoderm of the third pair of pharyngeal pouches and the surrounding mesenchyme. Recent experimental studies indicate that cells of neural crest origin are also involved in the development of the thymus.

17. **C** Clefts of the posterior or secondary palate result from failure of the mesenchymal masses in the lateral palatine processes to meet with each other and the nasal septum. Such clefts extend through the soft and hard palates and are located posterior to the incisive fossa. Clefts anterior to the incisive fossa are classified as clefts of the anterior or primary palate and result from failure of the mesenchymal masses in the lateral palatine processes to meet and fuse with the mesenchyme in the primary palate. Cleft palate and cleft lip are caused by genetic and environmental factors (multifactorial inheritance).

18. **D** The cartilage of the third pharyngeal arch ossifies to form the greater cornu and the inferior part of the hyoid bone. The other derivative of this pharyngeal arch is the stylopharyngeus muscle. The skeletal and muscular derivatives of the other pharyngeal arches are many.

19. **B** The nasolacrimal duct develops from a cordlike thickening of ectoderm in the floor of the groove between the maxillary and lateral nasal prominences. Connection of the lacrimal sac of the eye with the nasal cavity allows tears to drain into the inferior meatus. Failure of the cordlike thickening of ectoderm to canalize results in atresia of the nasolacrimal duct, the most common disorder of the lacrimal apparatus. Unilateral clefting of the upper lip results from failure of the maxillary prominence on the affected side to merge with the medial nasal prominence on the same side. The intermaxillary segment of the upper jaw is formed by the fusion of the medial nasal prominences. Cleft lip occurs more frequently in males, with an incidence of about 1 in 1000 live births.

Answers and Explanations *Continued*

20. **D** The primary palate develops from the intermaxillary segment of the maxilla (the merged medial nasal prominences). It represents a relatively small part of the adult hard palate. The lateral palatine processes (or lateral palatal processes) begin to develop in the sixth week from the maxillary prominences. Fusion of the lateral palatine processes with each other in the median plane, and with the primary palate anteriorly, begins during the ninth week and is completed by the 12th week.

21. **A** The external acoustic meatus develops from the first pharyngeal groove. The remaining three pharyngeal grooves become obliterated by the second pharyngeal arch, which grows over them as the neck develops. The first pharyngeal pouch gives rise to the tympanic cavity, mastoid antrum, and pharyngotympanic tube. The second pharyngeal pouch gives rise to the palatine tonsil.

22. **E** Clefting of the upper lip is a relatively common congenital anomaly with an incidence of about 1 in 1000 live births. It occurs more commonly in males. Cleft lip may be unilateral or bilateral and results from a failure of the maxillary prominence to merge with the medial nasal prominence. Although cleft lip and cleft palate frequently occur together, the embryological basis of cleft lip is distinct from that of cleft palate. Cleft lip is a multifactorial disorder with both genetic and environmental factors involved. Surgical closure of a cleft lip is usually done when the infant is about 2 months old.

23. **A** Failure of the lateral palatine processes to fuse with the primary palate results in a primary cleft palate (anterior cleft anomaly). It is located anterior to the incisive fossa. When the lateral palatine processes fail to meet and fuse in the midline, the resulting condition is described as a posterior cleft anomaly. This defect is located posterior to the incisive fossa, and occurs more commonly in females. Surgical closure of the palate is usually performed before the child reaches 1 year of age.

24. **A** The first pharyngeal groove gives rise to the external acoustic meatus. The remaining three (second, third, and fourth) pharyngeal grooves normally become obliterated by the second pharyngeal arch, which overgrows them. A transient ectoderm-lined cervical sinus is formed, which may persist as a lateral cervical (branchial) cyst. Failure of the pharyngeal grooves to involute is usually located at the angle of the mandible, anterior to the sternocleidomastoid muscle. It may appear at any age, but usually in young adults. Accessory thyroid tissue, thyroglossal duct cyst, and dermoid cyst are found in the midline of the neck. They usually are diagnosed at birth or within the first few years of life. The CT scan findings make the diagnosis of a swollen lymph node unlikely.

■ FIVE-CHOICE ASSOCIATION QUESTIONS

Directions: Each group of questions below consists of a numbered list of descriptive words or phrases accompanied by a diagram with certain parts indicated by letters or by a list of lettered headings. For each numbered word or phrase, **select the lettered part or heading** that matches it correctly and then insert the letter in the space to the right of the appropriate number. Sometimes more than one numbered word or phrase may be correctly matched to the same lettered part or heading.

Five-Choice Association Questions *Continued*

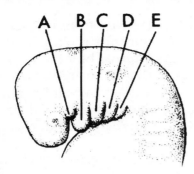

1. _____ Supplied by the vagus nerve
2. _____ Its cartilage forms the stapes
3. _____ Forms inferior part of the face
4. _____ Gives rise to the lateral palatine process
5. _____ Its muscle element gives rise to the platysma
6. _____ Its cartilage forms a greater cornu of the hyoid bone

A. First pharyngeal arch
B. Second pharyngeal arch
C. Third pharyngeal arch

D. Fourth pharyngeal arch
E. Sixth pharyngeal arch

7. _____ Glossopharyngeal nerve
8. _____ Muscles of facial expression
9. _____ Supplied by the maxillary division of the fifth cranial nerve
10. _____ Stylohyoid ligament
11. _____ Superior laryngeal branch of the vagus nerve
12. _____ Meckel cartilage
13. _____ Gives rise to the lateral palatine process
14. _____ Greater cornu of the hyoid bone
15. _____ Forms lateral part of the upper lip
16. _____ Lesser cornua of the hyoid bone
17. _____ Main contributor of the thyroid cartilage
18. _____ Supplied by CN X

19. _____ Becomes the external acoustic meatus
20. _____ Becomes the inferior parathyroid gland
21. _____ Tubotympanic recess
22. _____ Gives rise to the ultimobranchial body
23. _____ Forms half of the thymus
24. _____ Gives rise to the pharyngotympanic tube

A. First pharyngeal pouch
B. Second pharyngeal pouch
C. Third pharyngeal pouch

D. Fourth pharyngeal pouch
E. Fifth pharyngeal pouch

25. _____ Thymus
26. _____ Superior parathyroid gland
27. _____ Inferior parathyroid gland
28. _____ May not develop

29. _____ Palatine tonsil
30. _____ Tubotympanic recess
31. _____ Internal branchial sinus
32. _____ Thyrocalcitonin

Five-Choice Association Questions *Continued*

33. _____ Derived from the second and third pharyngeal arch cartilages
34. _____ Internal branchial sinus
35. _____ Derived from the second pharyngeal groove and cervical sinus
36. _____ External branchial sinus
37. _____ Internal and external carotid arteries
38. _____ Organ derived from the second pharyngeal pouch and mesenchyme

---

■ ANSWERS AND EXPLANATIONS

1. **E** The fourth pharyngeal arch is supplied by the superior laryngeal branch of the vagus nerve (CN X). This nerve supplies pharyngeal and laryngeal muscles that develop from the fourth arch.

2. **C** The dorsal end of the second arch cartilage (Reichert cartilage) ossifies to form the stapes of the middle ear and the styloid process of the temporal bone. The ventral ends of the cartilages give rise to the lesser cornua and superior part of the body of the hyoid bone. The perichondrium of this cartilage forms the stylohyoid ligament.

3. **B** The mandibular prominences of the first pharyngeal arches form the inferior part of the face. The mandible develops in these prominences by intramembranous bone formation around the first arch cartilages. The superior part of the face forms from the maxillary prominences of the first arches.

4. **A** The lateral palatine processes arise as horizontal mesenchymal projections from the inner surfaces of the maxillary prominences of the first pharyngeal arches. The lateral palatine processes grow toward each other and fuse.

5. **C** The muscle elements in the second pharyngeal arches give rise to myoblasts that migrate into the facial region and around the ears and eyes. These myoblasts differentiate into the muscles of facial expression.

6. **D** The third arch cartilages, located in the ventral portions of the arches, ossify to form the greater cornua and the inferior part of the body of the hyoid bone.

7. **C** The glossopharyngeal nerve (CN IX) is the nerve of the third pharyngeal arch; hence, it supplies the stylopharyngeus muscle derived from the muscle element in this arch. Because the dorsal part of the root of the tongue is derived from the third arch, its sensory innervation is partly supplied by the glossopharyngeal nerve.

8. **B** The muscles of facial expression are derived from the second pharyngeal arch. Other muscles derived from this arch are the stylohyoid, the posterior belly of the digastric, and the stapedius. From the position of the second arch in the embryo, one would not expect it to give rise to facial muscles. During development, the developing muscle cells (myoblasts) migrate to the head and retain their original nerve supply from the second arch (i.e., the facial nerve).

Answers and Explanations *Continued*

9. **A** The maxillary prominence of the first pharyngeal arch is supplied by the maxillary division of the trigeminal nerve (CN V). The mandibular prominence is supplied by the mandibular branch of this nerve. The trigeminal nerve also supplies the muscles of mastication and other muscles derived from this arch. This nerve also supplies the skin over the mandible and the anterior two thirds of the tongue.

10. **B** The stylohyoid ligament is derived from the perichondrium of the second pharyngeal arch cartilage, after it regresses between the styloid process and the hyoid bone.

11. **D** The superior laryngeal branch of the vagus nerve (CN X) supplies the fourth pharyngeal arch. Hence, it supplies the cricothyroid muscle and the constrictors of the pharynx that are derived from the muscle element in this arch.

12. **B** Meckel cartilage is the name given to the cartilage located in the mandibular process of the first pharyngeal arch. Its dorsal portion, related to the developing internal ear, becomes ossified to form two middle ear bones (malleus and incus).

13. **A** The internal parts of the maxillary prominences of the first pair of pharyngeal arches give rise to two horizontal projections called lateral palatine processes. These processes later fuse with each other and with the nasal septum to form the posterior or secondary palate. Incomplete fusion of these processes results in a cleft of the posterior palate.

14. **C** The greater cornua of the hyoid bone are derived from the cartilages of the third pair of pharyngeal arches. The inferior part of the body of this bone is also derived by endochondral ossification of the cartilages of these arches.

15. **A** The maxillary prominence of the first pharyngeal arch gives rise to the lateral part of the upper lip. It fuses with the intermaxillary segment (merged medial nasal prominences), which gives rise to the central portion or philtrum of the lip.

16. **B** The lesser cornua of the hyoid bone are derived from the cartilages of the second pharyngeal arches. The superior part of the body of this bone is also derived by endochondral ossification of these cartilages.

17. **D** The cartilaginous components of the fourth pair of pharyngeal arches give rise to large parts of the thyroid cartilage. The cartilages of the sixth arches are also main contributors.

18. **D** The fourth pharyngeal arch is supplied by the vagus nerve (CN X). This nerve supplies the intrinsic muscles of the larynx, which develop from myoblasts in the fourth arch.

19. **B** The external acoustic meatus develops from the dorsal end of the first pharyngeal groove. All other pharyngeal grooves normally disappear as the neck forms.

20. **D** The solid dorsal bulbar portion of the third pharyngeal pouch differentiates into an inferior parathyroid gland. These glands descend with the thymus gland and later leave it to lie on the posterior surface of the thyroid gland.

21. **C** The tubotympanic recess becomes the pharyngotympanic tube, tympanic cavity, and antrum. Its epithelium forms the internal layer of the tympanic membrane.

22. **E** The ventral portions of the fourth pair of pharyngeal pouches give rise to the ultimobranchial bodies. If present, the fifth pair of pouches may also contribute to the formation of these bodies. The

Answers and Explanations *Continued*

ultimobranchial bodies later fuse with the thyroid gland and are represented by cells called C or parafollicular cells. These cells produce calcitonin, an important hormone concerned with calcium metabolism.

23. **A** The ventral portions of the third pair of pharyngeal pouches fuse and give rise to the primordium of the thymus. This thymic mass becomes invaded by mesenchymal cells that break up the gland into lobules. The thymic corpuscles (Hassall corpuscles) appear to be derived from the endodermal epithelium. The origin of the thymocytes is controversial, but they are believed to be mesenchymal.

24. **C** The tubotympanic recess gives rise to the epithelium and glands of the pharyngotympanic tube. The bony wall in its posterior third and the remaining cartilaginous wall are derived from the surrounding mesenchyme.

25. **C** The elongated ventral portions of the third pair of pharyngeal pouches migrate medially and fuse to form the primordium of the thymus. Development of the thymus is not complete at birth; it continues to grow and reaches its greatest size at puberty. Thereafter it becomes very small and is difficult to locate.

26. **D** The dorsal bulbar portion of each fourth pharyngeal pouch develops into a superior parathyroid gland. They come to lie on the dorsal surface of the thyroid gland.

27. **C** The dorsal bulbar portion of each third pharyngeal pouch differentiates into a parathyroid gland. These glands migrate caudally with the thymus, which develops from the ventral portions of this pair of pharyngeal pouches. Hence, the parathyroid glands derived from the third pair of pouches come to lie further caudally than those from the fourth pair of pouches. Because of this descent, some-

times the inferior parathyroid glands are located in other than their normal position; that is, they may be drawn into the thorax by the descent of the thymus.

28. **E** The fifth pair of pharyngeal pouches often do not develop. When present, they are rudimentary and incorporated into the fourth pair of pharyngeal pouches.

29. **B** The palatine tonsils are derived from the endoderm of the second pair of pharyngeal pouches and the associated mesenchyme. The endoderm of the pouches gives rise to the surface epithelium and the lining of the crypts of the tonsil. The mesenchyme around the developing crypts differentiates into lymphoid tissue.

30. **A** The epithelium and the glands of the pharyngotympanic tube are derived from the elongated tubotympanic recess, the expanded first pharyngeal pouch. This recess also gives rise to the tympanic cavity and antrum. The connective tissue and cartilaginous parts of the auditory tube are derived from the mesenchyme surrounding the tubotympanic recess.

31. **B** Internal branchial sinuses open into the pharynx. They commonly are derived from a remnant of the second pharyngeal pouch; hence, they typically open into the intratonsillar fossa, the remains of the opening into the second pharyngeal pouch.

32. **D** Calcitonin is produced by the parafollicular cells (C cells) of the thyroid gland, derived from the ultimobranchial bodies. These bodies develop from the ventral portions of the fourth pair of pharyngeal pouches. If the fifth pair of pouches develop, they may contribute to the formation of the ultimobranchial bodies.

33. **E** The hyoid bone develops by endochondral ossification of the ventral ends of the second and third pharyngeal arch

Answers and Explanations *Continued*

cartilages. The second arch cartilages give rise to the lesser cornua and the superior part of the body, and the third arch cartilages give rise to the greater cornua and the inferior part of the body of the hyoid bone.

34. **C** Internal branchial sinuses opening into the pharynx are rare. Because they almost always open into the intratonsillar fossa or near the palatopharyngeal arch, these sinuses usually result from partial persistence of part of the second pharyngeal pouch. These pouches commonly give rise to the epithelium and the lining of the crypts of the palatine tonsils.

35. **A** External branchial sinuses (also called lateral cervical sinuses) are uncommon. Almost all of those that open on the side of the neck result from failure of the second pharyngeal groove to obliterate. The sinuses typically open on the inferior one third of a line that runs from the auricle along the anterior border of the sterno-cleidomastoid muscle to the jugular notch. There often is an intermittent discharge of mucus from the opening, resulting from infection of the sinus.

36. **A** External branchial (lateral cervical) sinuses are lined with stratified squamous or columnar epithelium; they are surrounded by a muscular wall. Thus, by pulling the skin inferiorly, it is possible to palpate the firm sinus as it extends superiorly.

37. **B** Sinuses and fistulas ascend through the subcutaneous tissue and the platysma muscle and between the external and internal carotid arteries.

38. **D** The surface epithelium and the lining of the crypts of the palatine tonsils are derived from the endoderm of the second pair of pharyngeal pouches. The mesenchyme that surrounds the pouches differentiates into lymphoid tissue that soon becomes organized into lymph nodules.

The Respiratory System

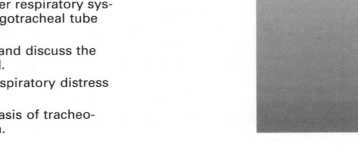

Objectives

Be able to:

- Describe the early development of the lower respiratory system, illustrating the formation of the laryngotracheal tube and its derivatives.
- List the four stages of lung development, and discuss the main events that occur during each period.
- Write a brief note on surfactant and the respiratory distress syndrome.
- Discuss and illustrate the embryological basis of tracheo-esophageal fistula with esophageal atresia.

■ FIVE-CHOICE COMPLETION QUESTIONS

Directions: Each of the following statements or questions is followed by five suggested responses or completions. **Select the one best answer** in each case.

1. The first indication of the lower respiratory tract in the human embryo is the laryngotracheal groove. It begins to develop in the primitive pharyngeal floor at _____ days.

   A. 19 to 21
   B. 22 to 24
   C. 25 to 27
   D. 28 to 30
   E. 31 to 33

2. The connective tissue, cartilage, and smooth muscle of the trachea are derived from the

   A. somatic mesoderm from the lateral plates
   B. splanchnic mesenchyme around the laryngotracheal tube
   C. endodermal lining of the laryngotracheal tube
   D. mesenchyme from the fourth to sixth pairs of pharyngeal arches
   E. neural crest

3. One eighth to one sixth of the adult number of alveoli are present in the lungs at birth. Their number increases after birth for at least _____ years.

   A. 2
   B. 4
   C. 6
   D. 8
   E. 10

Five-Choice Completion Questions *Continued*

4. Each of the following anomalies of the lower respiratory tract is uncommon *except*
   A. tracheal stenosis
   B. tracheal diverticulum
   C. tracheal atresia
   D. congenital emphysema
   E. tracheoesophageal fistula

5. Pulmonary surfactant is produced by
   A. type I alveolar epithelial cells
   B. blood cells
   C. alveolar macrophages (phagocytes)
   D. endothelial cells
   E. type II alveolar epithelial cells

6. Pulmonary surfactant begins to form in the human fetus at about _____ weeks.
   A. 16
   B. 20
   C. 24
   D. 28
   E. 32

7. A fetus born prematurely during which of the following periods of lung development may survive?
   A. organogenetic
   B. terminal sac
   C. pseudoglandular
   D. canalicular
   E. embryonic

8. The lungs at birth are about half inflated with liquid derived largely from the
   A. lung tissues
   B. nasal mucus
   C. amniotic fluid
   D. tracheal glands
   E. maternal blood

9. Hyaline membrane disease was suspected in a premature infant who showed signs of labored breathing and tachypnea at birth. This condition is caused by which of the following?
   A. deficiency of pulmonary surfactant
   B. excess pulmonary surfactant
   C. abnormal differentiation of type I alveolar cells
   D. intrauterine asphyxia
   E. atelectasis

10. Radiographic examination of an infant's lungs revealed areas of increased parenchymal density. A diagnosis of congenital lung cysts was made. The embryological basis of this defect involves which of the following?
    A. hypoplasia of the lungs
    B. deficiency of surfactant
    C. dilation of the terminal bronchi
    D. defective tracheoesophageal septum
    E. tracheal atresia

Five-Choice Completion Questions *Continued*

11. A large mass of nonfunctional lung tissue was seen in the chest radiograph of a young girl. A diagnosis of pulmonary sequestration (accessory lung tissue) was made. This condition is probably due to
    A. failure of a bronchial bud to develop
    B. deficiency of pulmonary surfactant
    C. disturbance in bronchial tree development
    D. a fistula between the trachea and esophagus
    E. abnormal development of an accessory lung bud

12. Regarding fetal breathing movements, all of the following are correct *except* that they
    A. occur periodically before birth
    B. facilitate exchange of oxygen and carbon dioxide between mother and fetus
    C. increase as the time of delivery approaches
    D. are essential for fetal lung development
    E. can be monitored before birth

■ ANSWERS AND EXPLANATIONS

1. **C** The median longitudinal laryngotracheal groove is recognizable at 26 to 27 days. As it deepens, its caudal end begins to separate from the foregut, giving rise to the tracheal and esophageal primordia. This division extends cranially until only the communication between the pharynx and the air passages (the laryngeal inlet) remains.

2. **B** The connective tissue, cartilage, and smooth muscle of the trachea and bronchi develop from splanchnic mesenchyme around the laryngotracheal tube. The striated muscles, cartilages, and connective tissues of the larynx are derived from mesenchyme of the fourth to sixth pairs of branchial arches.

3. **D** Alveolar production begins in the human lungs during the late fetal period, but characteristic pulmonary alveoli probably do not form until respiration begins. Alveoli continue to form until at least the eighth year. About 30 to 50 million alveoli are present at birth, and by the eighth year, about 300 million alveoli are present. The number of alveoli in the adult lung varies between 250 and 500 million.

4. **E** Tracheoesophageal fistula occurs about once in 2500 births, predominantly in males. This connection between the trachea and esophagus results from incomplete separation of the respiratory and digestive portions of the foregut. In most cases, there is also esophageal atresia.

5. **E** The type II alveolar epithelial cells are believed to produce surfactant, a surface-active agent. Surfactant forms a monomolecular layer over pulmonary alveolar surfaces and is capable of lowering surface tension at the air-alveolar interface when respiration begins at birth, thereby maintaining patency of the alveoli. Absence or deficiency of surfactant is a major cause of hyaline membrane disease.

Answers and Explanations *Continued*

6. **C** It is generally agreed that the type II cells of the epithelium of the alveoli, or secretory cells, begin to produce surfactant at about 24 weeks. It has been suggested that prolonged intrauterine asphyxia may produce reversible changes in these cells, making them incapable of producing surfactant. However, there are probably several causes for absence or deficiency of surfactant, particularly in premature infants.

7. **B** During the terminal sac period (24 weeks to birth), a fetus may survive if born prematurely, especially if it weighs 1000 gm or more. The terminal air sacs appear as outpouchings of the respiratory bronchioles and are soon surrounded by a rich capillary network. Before this time, the fetal lungs usually are incapable of providing adequate gas exchange, mainly because of inadequate pulmonary vasculature.

8. **A** The fluid in the lungs at birth is believed to be derived mainly from the lower respiratory tract itself. As much as 30 ml/day of fluid may be produced by the fetal tracheobronchial tree near term. The fluid in the lungs differs in composition from plasma, lymph, and amniotic fluid. Some of the liquid in the lungs probably comes from the tracheal glands, and some is probably amniotic fluid. It is well established that respiratory movements occur before birth, causing aspiration of amniotic fluid.

9. **A** Pulmonary surfactant, produced by type II alveolar cells, counteracts surface tension forces and facilitates expansion of the terminal sacs or primordial alveoli. Surfactant deficiency leads to hyaline membrane disease, a common cause of neonatal deaths, especially among infants born prematurely.

10. **C** Congenital lung cysts arise from abnormal development and dilation of the terminal bronchi. Because of air or fluid in the cysts, the lungs have a honeycomb appearance on radiographs.

11. **E** Pulmonary sequestration (accessory lung tissue) is an aberrant mass of nonfunctional lung tissue that does not communicate with the tracheobronchial tree. It is now believed that pulmonary sequestration, intralobular (in the lung) or extralobular (outside the lung), results from abnormal development of an accessory lung bud derived from the foregut of the embryo. This nonfunctional mass of pulmonary tissue is nourished by systemic arteries. Pulmonary sequestration is usually detected as an incidental finding on chest radiography or at surgery, and most are resected. Deficiency of pulmonary surfactant is associated with hyaline membrane disease. Failure of a bronchial bud to develop leads to agenesis of a lung. Tracheoesophageal fistula results from incomplete separation of the trachea and the esophagus during their development from the foregut.

12. **B** Periodic breathing movements occur in utero and cause aspiration of amniotic fluid into the lungs. Exchange of gases between mother and fetus occurs in the placenta before birth and in the lungs after birth. The fluid in the lungs is cleared at birth and replaced by gases with the infant's breathing. Prenatal breathing movements stimulate lung development. Fetal breathing movements can be detected and monitored by real-time ultrasonography. The pattern of fetal breathing movements is used for diagnosis of labor and for assessing fetal outcome in preterm delivery.

■ FIVE-CHOICE ASSOCIATION QUESTIONS

Directions: Each group of questions below consists of a numbered list of descriptive words or phrases accompanied by a diagram with certain parts indicated by letters or by a list of lettered headings. For each numbered word or phrase, **select the lettered part or heading** that matches it correctly and then insert the letter in the space to the right of the appropriate number. Sometimes more than one numbered word or phrase may be correctly matched to the same lettered part or heading.

1. _____ Lung bud
2. _____ Esophagus
3. _____ Divides the foregut into the laryngotracheal tube and esophagus
4. _____ Gives rise to the larynx, trachea, bronchi, and lungs
5. _____ Foregut
6. _____ Divides into bronchial buds

7. _____ Associated with polyhydramnios
8. _____ Derived from the lung bud
9. _____ Esophageal atresia
10. _____ Laryngotracheal fistula
11. _____ Allows air to enter the gastrointestinal tract

A. Laryngotracheal groove
B. Somatic mesoderm
C. Surfactant
D. Esophageal atresia
E. Splanchnic mesenchyme

12. _____ Polyhydramnios
13. _____ Tracheal cartilage
14. _____ Type II alveolar cells
15. _____ Tracheoesophageal fistula
16. _____ Prevents atelectasis
17. _____ Diverticulum of the pharynx
18. _____ Hyaline membrane disease
19. _____ Parietal pleura

20. _____ Primordium of the left lung
21. _____ Its glands are derived from the laryngotracheal tube
22. _____ Pericardioperitoneal canal
23. _____ Future right pleural cavity
24. _____ Splanchnic mesenchyme
25. _____ Will become the parietal pleura

■ ANSWERS AND EXPLANATIONS

1. **C** The lung bud develops at the caudal end of the laryngotracheal tube and soon divides into two bronchial buds. These buds differentiate into the bronchi and their ramifications in the lungs.

2. **B** The esophagus is derived from the foregut and separated from the laryngotracheal tube when the tracheoesophageal septum formed.

3. **D** The tracheoesophageal septum, formed by the gradual fusion of the tracheoesophageal folds, divides the foregut into the laryngotracheal tube and the esophagus. Incomplete separation of these structures results in one of the varieties of tracheoesophageal fistula.

4. **E** The endodermal lining of the laryngotracheal tube gives rise to the epithelium and glands of the larynx, trachea, and bronchi and to the pulmonary lining epithelium. The connective tissue, cartilage, and smooth muscle of these structures develop from the surrounding splanchnic mesenchyme.

5. **A** The foregut gives rise to the pharynx and its derivatives, the lower respiratory tract, esophagus, stomach, and first part of the duodenum as far as the entry of the bile duct, and to the liver and pancreas.

6. **C** The lung bud that forms at the caudal end of the laryngotracheal tube during the fourth week gives rise to two bronchial buds. These buds differentiate into the bronchi and their ramifications in the lungs.

7. **A** Polyhydramnios (excess amniotic fluid) is frequent in mothers of fetuses that have esophageal atresia because amniotic fluid cannot pass to the intestines for absorption and subsequent transfer to the placenta for disposal. If you selected choice **C**, you were partly right because

esophageal atresia often is associated with tracheoesophageal fistula. It must be understood that esophageal atresia may occur as a separate anomaly and that tracheoesophageal fistula without esophageal atresia also occurs. With an isolated fistula, polyhydramnios probably would not be present because amniotic fluid could pass to the stomach and intestines.

8. **D** The bronchi are derived from divisions of the lung bud called bronchial (lung) buds. These buds differentiate into the bronchi and their ramifications in the lungs.

9. **A** Atresia or lack of continuity of the esophagus may be encountered as a separate congenital anomaly. Esophageal atresia commonly is associated with tracheoesophageal fistula. An overall incidence of these associated anomalies of 1 in 2500 neonates is accepted. About two thirds of the cases occur in males. Infants present with excessive saliva, gagging, vomiting if fed, and cyanosis. Aspiration of gastric contents is responsible for the severe pulmonary symptoms.

10. **C** The type of tracheoesophageal fistula shown is the most common (more than 85% of cases). The fistula results from incomplete fusion of tracheoesophageal folds. This canal forms at the site of the defective tracheoesophageal septum and permits communication between the esophagus and trachea. The commonly associated esophageal atresia probably results from incomplete recanalization of the upper part of the esophagus.

11. **C** In the usual type of tracheoesophageal fistula, associated with the inferior end of the esophageal atresia, there is a fistulous connection between the lower esophagus and the trachea (as shown). Not only does this fistula allow gastric contents to enter the lungs, causing severe pulmonary symptoms, but it permits air to enter the gastrointestinal tract. As a

Answers and Explanations *Continued*

result, the abdomen rapidly becomes distended and the intestines promptly fill with air.

12. **D** An excess of amniotic fluid commonly is associated with esophageal atresia and tracheoesophageal fistula because amniotic fluid cannot pass to the intestines for absorption and subsequent transfer to the placenta for disposal. Polyhydramnios may also be associated with meroanencephaly (partial absence of the brain), possibly because the fetus lacks the neural control for swallowing amniotic fluid.

13. **E** The tracheal cartilages develop from the splanchnic mesenchyme that surrounds the laryngotracheal tube. This mesenchyme also gives rise to the connective tissue and smooth muscle of the trachea.

14. **C** The type II alveolar cells, the secretory cells of the lining epithelium, produce the surface-active agent called surfactant. These cells are believed to begin producing surfactant at about 24 weeks.

15. **D** A tracheoesophageal fistula (connection between the trachea and esophagus) occurs about once in 2500 births, predominantly in males. In 85 per cent of cases, this anomaly is associated with esophageal atresia.

16. **C** Surfactant, a substance produced by the type II alveolar cells, is capable of lowering the surface tension at the air-alveolar surface, thereby maintaining patency of the alveoli and preventing atelectasis (imperfect expansion or collapse of the lungs).

17. **A** The longitudinal laryngotracheal groove is a diverticulum of the endodermal floor of the primitive pharynx, caudal to the hypobranchial eminence (pri-

mordium of the posterior one third of the tongue and of the epiglottis). The endodermal lining of this groove gives rise to the epithelium and glands of the larynx, trachea, and bronchi and to the pulmonary lining epithelium.

18. **C** Hyaline membrane disease, a common cause of death in the perinatal period, is associated with an absence or deficiency of surfactant (a surface tension–lowering agent). In this disease, which occurs particularly in babies born prematurely, a membrane-like structure lines the respiratory bronchioles, alveolar ducts, and alveoli. Because of the deficiency of surfactant, there is a tendency for the alveoli to collapse (atelectasis).

19. **B** The parietal pleura develops from the mesoderm that lines the thoracic body wall. As the lungs invaginate the pericardioperitoneal cavities (primitive pleural cavities), the space between the parietal and visceral layers of pleura is reduced to a narrow interval.

20. **D** The left bronchial bud, together with the surrounding splanchnic mesenchyme, gives rise to the left lung. At the stage shown, the bronchial buds represent the two lobes of the left lung.

21. **B** The endodermal lining of the middle portion of the laryngotracheal tube gives rise to the epithelium and glands of the trachea. The cartilage, connective tissue, and smooth muscle are derived from the surrounding splanchnic mesenchyme.

22. **A** The pericardioperitoneal canal connects the pericardial cavity and the peritoneal cavity during the fourth and fifth weeks. After division of the intraembryonic coelom into three separate cavities, these canals become the pleural cavities.

23. **A** The future right pleural cavity is represented by the right pericardioperito-

Answers and Explanations *Continued*

neal canal. The developing lungs grow into the splanchnic mesoderm of the medial walls of the pericardioperitoneal canals.

24. **C** The splanchnic mesenchyme surrounding the developing lungs gives rise to the bronchial musculature and cartilaginous rings and to the pulmonary connective tissue and capillaries. The splanchnic mesenchyme also gives rise to the visceral pleura covering the lungs.

25. **E** The pleural cavities are lined externally by a layer of somatic mesoderm; this layer subsequently becomes the parietal pleura. The invagination of the lungs into the developing pleural cavities is so complete that the space between the visceral and parietal layers of pleura becomes greatly reduced.

■ NOTES

The Digestive System 12

Objectives

Be able to:

- Construct and label diagrams illustrating the formation of the primordial gut by the incorporation of the dorsal part of the yolk sac into the embryo.
- List the derivatives of the foregut.
- Describe the rotation of the stomach and formation of the omental bursa (lesser sac of peritoneum).
- Describe the development of the duodenum, liver, biliary apparatus, pancreas, and spleen.
- List the derivatives of the midgut, and illustrate herniation, rotation, reduction, and fixation of the midgut.
- Write brief notes on pyloric stenosis, omphalocele, incomplete rotation and volvulus of the midgut, intestinal stenosis and atresia, and Meckel diverticulum.
- List the derivatives of the hindgut.
- Describe partitioning of the cloaca.
- Describe development of the anal canal, and write short notes on imperforate anus and anorectal agenesis with fistula.

■ FIVE-CHOICE COMPLETION QUESTIONS

Directions: Each of the following statements or questions is followed by five suggested responses or completions. **Select the one best answer** in each case.

1. As the stomach acquires its adult shape, it rotates around its longitudinal axis. Which of the following events does not result from this rotation?

    A. Ventral border of the stomach moves to the right.
    B. Dorsal border of the stomach moves to the left.
    C. Dorsal mesogastrium is carried to the left.
    D. Dorsal part of the stomach grows rapidly.
    E. Duodenum slowly rotates to the right.

2. Derivatives of the caudal portion of the embryonic foregut are mainly supplied by which of the following arteries?

    A. superior mesenteric
    B. inferior mesenteric
    C. gastro-omental
    D. celiac
    E. right gastric

Five-Choice Completion Questions *Continued*

3. Each of the following statements about the developing duodenum is true *except*
   A. It is a derivative of the foregut and midgut.
   B. The yolk stalk is attached to the apex of the duodenal loop.
   C. It is supplied by branches of the foregut and midgut arteries.
   D. It becomes C-shaped as the stomach rotates.
   E. Its lumen is temporarily obliterated by epithelial cells.

4. Hematopoiesis begins in the liver during the _____ week.
   A. third
   B. fourth
   C. fifth
   D. sixth
   E. seventh

5. The most common type of anorectal anomaly is
   A. anal stenosis
   B. ectopic anus
   C. anorectal agenesis
   D. anal agenesis
   E. persistent anal membrane

6. The anal membrane usually ruptures at the end of the _____ week.
   A. fifth
   B. sixth
   C. seventh
   D. eighth
   E. ninth

7. Pyloric stenosis is characterized by vomiting, usually starting in the second or third week after birth. The narrowing of the pyloric lumen results primarily from
   A. hypertrophy of the longitudinal muscular layer
   B. a diaphragm-like narrowing of the pyloric lumen
   C. hypertrophy of the circular muscular layer
   D. persistence of the solid stage of pyloric development
   E. a so-called fetal vascular accident in the pylorus

8. The junction of the endodermal epithelium of the hindgut and the ectodermal epithelium of the proctodeum or anal pit is believed to be indicated by the
   A. pectinate line
   B. levator ani muscle
   C. white line
   D. external sphincter
   E. superior ends of the anal columns

Five-Choice Completion Questions *Continued*

9. All the following statements about an ileal or Meckel diverticulum are true *except:*
   A. It is a common anomaly of the small intestine.
   B. It may become a leading point for an intussusception.
   C. Hemorrhage is a common sign of it during infancy.
   D. It is located on the mesenteric side of the ileum.
   E. Gastric mucosa is the most common ectopic tissue in it.

10. Anorectal agenesis is more common in males than in females and is usually associated with a rectourethral fistula. The embryologic basis of the fistula is
    A. failure of the proctodeum to develop
    B. agenesis of the urorectal septum
    C. failure of fixation of the hindgut
    D. abnormal partitioning of the cloaca
    E. premature rupture of the anal membrane

11. A 3-week-old infant has a history of projectile vomiting. The vomitus did not contain bile. The child cried a lot and was constantly hungry but did not gain any weight. Which of the following conditions would best account for these symptoms?
    A. Meckel diverticulum
    B. esophageal atresia
    C. hypertrophic pyloric stenosis
    D. duodenal atresia
    E. tracheoesophageal fistula

12. Massive rectal bleeding was observed in an infant. The color of the blood ranged from bright to dark red. The child appeared to be free of any pain. A diagnosis of Meckel diverticulum was made. This condition is associated with which of the following?
    A. remnant of the yolk stalk
    B. duplication of the intestine
    C. subhepatic cecum and appendix
    D. nonrotation of the midgut
    E. herniation of the intestines

13. Esophageal atresia was diagnosed in a newborn with symptoms of excessive salivation and almost instant vomiting of food. This congenital defect may be associated with each of the following *except*
    A. oligohydramnios
    B. posterior deviation of the tracheoesophageal septum
    C. a defective tracheoesophageal septum
    D. prematurity
    E. fistula to the trachea

Five-Choice Completion Questions *Continued*

14. Recanalization of the esophagus occurs during _____ week of development.
    A. fourth
    B. sixth
    C. eighth
    D. tenth
    E. twelfth

15. All of the following statements about the omental bursa are correct *except* that it
    A. develops in the mesenchyme of the dorsal mesogastrium
    B. develops in the mesenchyme of the ventral mesentery
    C. communicates with the peritoneal cavity
    D. facilitates movement of the stomach
    E. is a potential site for abscess formation

16. The ventral mesentery of the foregut gives rise to which of the following?
    A. lesser omentum
    B. falciform ligament
    C. visceral peritoneum of the liver
    D. all of the above
    E. none of the above

17. Extrahepatic biliary atresia was diagnosed in a newborn infant. Regarding this congenital defect, which of the following statements is (are) correct?
    A. It results from a failure of the biliary ducts to canalize.
    B. It occurs in about 1 in 10,000 to 1 in 15,000 live births.
    C. This is the most serious anomaly of the extrahepatic biliary system.
    D. Liver infection during late fetal development may result in extrahepatic biliary atresia.
    E. All of the above

■ ANSWERS AND EXPLANATIONS

1. **D**   Growth of the stomach occurs during rotation, but it does not result from it. The faster growth of the original dorsal part of the stomach gives rise to the greater curvature of the stomach. Rotation of the stomach explains why the left vagus nerve supplies the anterior wall of the adult stomach and why the right vagus innervates its posterior wall.

2. **D**   The celiac artery supplies derivatives of the caudal part of the embryonic foregut. It arises from the anterior aspect of the aorta just inferior to the aortic hiatus. It divides into the left gastric, hepatic, and splenic arteries, which supply most of the foregut derivatives (inferior part of the esophagus, stomach, superior part of the duodenum, liver, pancreas, and biliary apparatus). If you chose **C** or **E**, you selected a correct answer because they supply some foregut derivatives. **D** is the best answer, however, because it provides the main blood supply to the caudal part of the foregut.

3. **B**   The yolk stalk (vitelline duct) is attached to the apex of the midgut loop

Answers and Explanations *Continued*

(future terminal part of ileum). The junction of the foregut and midgut parts of the duodenum is located just distal to the point of entrance of the bile duct (common bile duct). Failure of the duodenum to recanalize results in stenosis (narrowing) or atresia (blockage) of the duodenum. Atresia occurs about twice as often as stenosis. Infants with duodenal atresia usually vomit green fluid because of the presence of bile. If the obstruction is superior to the point of entrance of the bile duct, the vomitus is not stained with bile.

4. **D** Hematopoiesis (blood formation) begins in the mesenchyme of the yolk sac and allantois during the third week, but it does not begin in the embryonic mesenchyme until early in the sixth week. Hematopoiesis occurs chiefly in the liver and spleen. Later, blood formation occurs in bone marrow and lymph nodes, in which sites it continues after birth.

5. **C** In most anorectal anomalies, the rectum ends superior to the anal canal and levator ani muscles. There usually is a fistulous connection with the urethra in males and the vagina in females. These defects produce intestinal obstruction because the fistulas seldom provide an adequate escape for gas and meconium (dark green fecal material).

6. **C** The anal membrane usually ruptures at the end of the seventh week. Imperforate anus resulting from failure of the anal membrane to perforate is uncommon. This type of imperforate anus consists of a septal occlusion of an otherwise normal anal canal. Some form of imperforate anus, usually anorectal agenesis, occurs about once in 5000 births and is much more common in males than in females. The reason for this sex difference is not known.

7. **C** Pyloric stenosis is common, especially in males (about 1 in 150). The pylorus is elongated and thickened to as much as twice its usual size. Forceful peristaltic waves of the gastric wall may be observed. The cause of pyloric stenosis is unknown, but hereditary factors are certainly involved. An acquired factor also appears to be involved in the pathogenesis of this "tumor," but its nature is unknown.

8. **A** The former site of the anal membrane, and thus the junction of the hindgut and the anal pit (proctodeum), is believed to be indicated by the irregular pectinate line (*pectin,* Latin for comb). The anal valves are attached along this line. Because of the different origins of the superior and inferior parts of the anal canal, the blood and nerve supply of the two parts differ. The inferior part of the anal canal, inferior to the pectinate line, is supplied by somatic sensory cutaneous fibers that respond immediately to painful stimuli, such as the prick of a needle. Thus, injection of a hemorrhoidal vein in the therapy of internal hemorrhoids is given superior to the pectinate line, where the mucosa is relatively insensitive to pain.

9. **D** Diverticula of the ileum, usually called Meckel diverticula, are always on the antimesenteric border of the ileum because they represent a persistent portion of the yolk stalk (vitelline duct), which attaches to the ventral side of the midgut loop. If a Meckel diverticulum inverts, it may serve as a leading point for intussusception (inversion of the diverticulum and ileum into the lumen of the ileum). Bleeding of a diverticulum arises from the peptic ulcer in or adjacent to the ectopic gastric mucosa, usually at the neck of the diverticulum.

10. **D** The urorectal septum, a mesenchymal septum or wedge between the allantois and the hindgut, typically grows caudally and fuses with the cloacal membrane. This partition divides the clo-

Answers and Explanations *Continued*

aca into the rectum dorsally and the urogenital sinus ventrally. Failure of the lateral infoldings of the cloaca, produced by caudal extensions of the urorectal septum, to fuse completely at all levels results in communication between the rectum and the urogenital sinus. The urogenital sinus in males gives rise to the urinary bladder and almost all the urethra. Thus, the fistula connects the rectum with the bladder (rectourethral fistula). In females, the urogenital sinus also gives rise to the vagina; rectovaginal fistulas are most commonly associated with anorectal agenesis in females.

11. **C**   Congenital hypertrophic pyloric stenosis involves an increase in the size of the circular muscle of the pylorus. This results in severe narrowing of the pyloric canal and obstruction to the passage of food. The infant expels the contents of the stomach with considerable (projectile) force. Males are affected more than females (5:1), and the cause is unknown. Blockage or atresia of the duodenum is associated with vomiting within a few hours of birth, and the vomitus usually contains bile.

12. **A**   The remnant of the proximal portion of the yolk stalk represents a Meckel diverticulum. It is the most frequent anomaly of the gastrointestinal tract and three to five times more prevalent in males than in females. Inflammation of the diverticulum can mimic the symptoms of acute appendicitis. The heterotopic gastric mucosa in the wall of the diverticulum may also cause bleeding from peptic ulceration. Other complications of Meckel diverticulum may be related to its connection with the umbilicus, leading to a volvulus or torsion of intestinal loops.

13. **A**   The fetus with esophageal atresia is unable to swallow amniotic fluid, resulting in an excess of amniotic fluid or polyhydramnios. In more than 85 per cent of cases, esophageal atresia is associated with a tracheoesophageal fistula. This communication between the trachea and esophagus is formed because of incomplete fusion of the tracheoesophageal folds. During the division of the foregut to form the laryngotracheal tube and esophagus, the tracheoesophageal septum may deviate in a posterior direction, resulting in an esophageal atresia. About one third of affected infants are born prematurely.

14. **C**   In the early embryo, the epithelial lining of the esophagus proliferates and partly or completely obliterates its lumen. During the eighth week, recanalization of the esophagus normally occurs and establishes the continuity of its lumen. Some isolated cases of esophageal atresia have been associated with a failure of recanalization of the esophagus. This condition has been attributed to defective growth of endodermal cells. Incomplete recanalization of the esophagus during the eighth week may lead to stenosis of the esophagus.

15. **B**   The omental bursa develops from isolated clefts in the mesenchyme of the dorsal mesentery. These clefts coalesce, forming the primordium of the omental bursa. The omental bursa (lesser sac) communicates with the main part of the peritoneal cavity through a small opening, the omental (epiploic) foramen. The omental bursa is located posterior to the stomach, and it permits the stomach to move freely as well as to change its size and shape. Clinically, the omental bursa is a potential site for the spread of infection and abscess formation.

16. **D**   The ventral mesentery of the foregut contributes to the formation of the lesser omentum (hepatogastric ligament), which passes from the liver to the lesser curvature of the stomach, and to the falciform ligament, which is a fold of peritoneum extending from the liver to the ventral abdominal wall. The peritoneal covering of the liver is also derived from

the ventral mesentery. The bile duct lies in the free margin of the lesser omentum, and the umbilical vein traverses the free border of the falciform ligament. Clinically, it is important to know the location of the bile duct and the umbilical vein.

17. **E** All of the statements are correct. The extrahepatic biliary system becomes occluded in the early embryo because of proliferation of endodermal cells. Later, it is canalized. Biliary atresia is an extremely serious developmental defect that requires surgical correction (portoenterostomy). When biliary atresia cannot be corrected surgically, the child may die if a liver transplantation is not performed. The 5-year survival for such patients is about 70 per cent. Surgical correction of atresia involving the distal portion of the extrahepatic duct has a better prognosis than atresia of the proximal or the entire extrahepatic duct system.

■ FIVE-CHOICE ASSOCIATION QUESTIONS

Directions: Each group of questions below consists of a numbered list of descriptive words or phrases accompanied by a diagram with certain parts indicated by letters or by a list of lettered headings. For each numbered word or phrase, **select the lettered part or heading** that matches it correctly and then insert the letter in the space to the right of the appropriate number. Sometimes more than one numbered word or phrase may be correctly matched to the same lettered part or heading.

A. Spleen
B. Yolk stalk
C. Gallbladder
D. Vermiform appendix
E. Celiac artery

1. _____ Primarily involved in extrahepatic biliary atresia
2. _____ Forms the major portion of the pancreas
3. _____ Penetrates the septum transversum
4. _____ Partly derived from the midgut
5. _____ Forms the inferior part of the head of the pancreas
6. _____ Extends into the dorsal mesentery

7. _____ Derived from the midgut loop
8. _____ Continuous with the apex of the midgut loop
9. _____ Organ derived solely from mesenchyme
10. _____ Derived from foregut
11. _____ Supplies foregut derivatives
12. _____ Umbilical sinus

A. Pyloric stenosis
B. Anorectal agenesis
C. Esophageal atresia
D. Omphalocele
E. Polyhydramnios

13. _____ Derived from the foregut and mid-gut
14. _____ Hepatoduodenal ligament
15. _____ Arises as a diverticulum of the foregut
16. _____ Visceral peritoneum
17. _____ Its free border contains the umbilical vein
18. _____ Embryonic site of hematopoiesis

19. _____ Faulty partitioning of foregut
20. _____ Herniation of intestines
21. _____ Causes projectile vomiting
22. _____ Duodenal obstruction
23. _____ Most common anomaly
24. _____ Faulty partitioning of cloaca

■ ANSWERS AND EXPLANATIONS

1. **B** In extrahepatic biliary atresia, parts of the hepatic ducts and the bile duct are not canalized. Portions of the bile ducts are blocked (atresia); other parts may have narrow lumina (stenosis). These severe anomalies are not common. The extrahepatic system of ducts develops as solid cords that typically soon become canalized. When this fails to occur, atresia results. If the lumen forms but is small, stenosis is present. Congenital atresia of the bile ducts may be caused by noxious agents acting during the development of the bile duct system. There is little evidence that this anomaly is hereditary; it rarely occurs in siblings (brothers or sisters). Jaundice gradually increases after birth; the stools are clay-colored, and the urine is dark brown. Can you explain the basis of these observations? See the text.

2. **D** The dorsal pancreatic bud forms the major portion of the pancreas; the inferior part of the head of the pancreas and the uncinate process are derived from the ventral pancreatic bud. The main pancreatic duct forms by fusion of the ducts of both pancreatic buds.

3. **C** The liver arises as a bud from the caudal part of the foregut late in the third week. This hepatic diverticulum extends ventrally and cranially into the mesenchyme of the septum transversum between the pericardial cavity and the yolk stalk. Subsequently, the liver lies between the layers of the ventral mesentery. These layers become the peritoneal covering of the liver and the ligaments associated with the liver.

4. **E** The epithelium and glands of the duodenum distal to the point of entrance of the bile duct are derived from the midgut. Other layers of the mucous membrane and the wall of the duodenum are derived from mesenchyme adjacent to the endodermal midgut. The epithelium and glands of the duodenum cranial to the entrance of this duct are derived from the foregut.

Answers and Explanations *Continued*

5. **A** The ventral pancreatic bud forms the inferior part of the head of the pancreas, including the uncinate process. Most of the pancreas develops from the dorsal bud. Sometimes the two pancreatic buds form a ring of pancreatic tissue around the duodenum (anular pancreas), which may cause obstruction of the duodenum.

6. **D** The dorsal pancreatic bud from the caudal end of the foregut appears slightly before the ventral pancreatic bud. As it grows, it extends into the dorsal mesentery. During rotation and growth of the duodenum, the ventral bud is carried dorsally with the bile duct and, subsequently, fuses with the dorsal bud.

7. **D** The vermiform appendix is derived from the cecal diverticulum, an outpouching from the antimesenteric side of the midgut loop. The distal end of the cecum does not grow rapidly; thus, the appendix forms. At birth, the appendix is relatively longer than in the adult and continuous with the apex of the cecum.

8. **B** The yolk stalk is attached to the apex of the midgut loop. The other end of this stalk is attached to the remnant of the yolk sac, located near the placenta. The yolk stalk normally degenerates at the end of the embryonic period, but in about 2 per cent of people, the proximal part of it persists as an ileal or Meckel diverticulum.

9. **A** The spleen is derived from a condensation of mesenchymal cells between the layers of the dorsal mesogastrium. The splenic artery is a branch of the foregut (celiac) artery; this explains why it gives off pancreatic branches, short gastric arteries, and the left gastro-omental artery. Recall that the stomach and pancreas are foregut derivatives.

10. **C** The gallbladder is derived from the foregut. The hepatic diverticulum from the foregut divides into two parts; the larger cranial part gives rise to the liver, and the caudal part gives rise to the gallbladder.

11. **E** The celiac artery carries blood from the aorta to the foregut derivatives (inferior end of the esophagus, stomach, liver, part of the duodenum, gallbladder, and part of the pancreas). The celiac artery also supplies the spleen, which develops from mesenchyme in the dorsal mesentery of the stomach.

12. **B** An umbilical sinus represents a remnant of the distal portion of the yolk stalk at the umbilicus. A remnant of the proximal portion of the yolk stalk is much more common and gives rise to a Meckel diverticulum. Umbilical sinuses are lined by intestinal mucosa and secrete a mucoid material. They may be attached to the ileum by a fibrous cord (a remnant of the proximal portion of the yolk stalk).

13. **B** The duodenum is derived from the caudal part of the foregut and the cranial part of the midgut. The junction of the foregut and midgut is at the apex of the embryonic duodenal loop and indicated in the adult by the point of entrance of the bile duct. Because of its dual origin, the duodenum is supplied by both the foregut (celiac) and midgut (superior mesenteric) arteries.

14. **A** The ventral mesentery between the cranial or superior part of the duodenum and the liver persists and gives rise to the hepatoduodenal ligament. The remainder of the ventral mesentery of the foregut gives rise to the hepatogastric ligament,

Answers and Explanations *Continued*

peritoneal covering of the liver, falciform ligament, and coronary and triangular ligaments of the liver. The superior part of the duodenum is the only part of the intestines that has a ventral mesentery.

15. **D** The liver arises as a bud or diverticulum from the caudal end of the foregut. The proliferating endodermal cells give rise to interlacing cords of cells, which become the liver parenchyma. The fibrous and hematopoietic tissue are derived from splanchnic mesenchyme.

16. **C** The visceral peritoneum of the liver is continuous with the hepatoduodenal ligament. This peritoneum is also continuous with the hepatogastric and falciform ligaments.

17. **E** The umbilical vein passes in the inferior free border of the falciform ligament on its way to the liver with well-oxygenated blood from the placenta. Within the liver, the umbilical vein is broken up by the proliferating hepatic cords. The hepatic sinusoids are derived from remnants of the umbilical and vitelline veins. The adult derivative of the extrahepatic portion of the umbilical vein is the ligamentum teres (round ligament) of the liver.

18. **D** The liver is an important site of blood formation in the embryo and early fetus. Hematopoiesis begins in the liver during the sixth week; before this, blood formation takes place in the extraembryonic mesenchyme of the yolk sac and allantois. Blood is later formed in the spleen, bone marrow, and lymph nodes. Blood formation continues after birth in the latter two sites.

19. **C** Esophageal atresia may occur as an isolated anomaly resulting from failure of canalization of the esophagus, but most often, it is associated with tracheoesophageal fistula. In more than 85 per cent of cases of this type of fistula, the esophagus ends blindly. The fistula between the inferior end of the esophagus and the trachea results from faulty or incomplete partitioning of the foregut into the esophagus and the laryngotracheal tube. Incomplete formation of the tracheoesophageal septum at any level may give rise to a fistula.

20. **D** Omphalocele is a congenital protrusion or herniation of the intestines through a large defect in the anterior abdominal wall at the umbilicus. This anomaly is believed to result from failure of the intestines to return from the umbilical cord during the 10th week. The hernial mass is covered by a thin, transparent membrane composed of peritoneum internally and amnion externally (from the amniotic covering of the umbilical cord).

21. **A** Pyloric stenosis (narrowing of the distal opening of the stomach) results from hypertrophy of the muscle fibers of the pylorus, principally the circular musculature. The typical clinical picture is an infant who appears normal at birth, but within a week or more, there is a gradual onset of vomiting that progresses to a projectile type.

22. **E** High intestinal obstruction (e.g., duodenal atresia) frequently is an accompaniment of polyhydramnios. Excessive amniotic fluid is also associated with meroanencephaly (partial absence of the brain) and esophageal atresia. With meroanencephaly, there appears to be difficulty in swallowing. In esophageal and duodenal atresia, amniotic fluid accumulates because it is unable to pass to the intestines for absorption.

23. **A** Pyloric stenosis is the most common of all the anomalies listed. It affects male infants much more often than female infants. An incidence of 1 in 500 births represents an approximate overall average. It affects 1 in every 150 males.

24. **B** Fistulas are associated with most cases of anorectal agenesis. The fistulas usually are rectourethral in males and rectovaginal in females. Anorectal agenesis with a fistula results from faulty or incomplete partitioning of the cloaca by the urorectal septum into the rectum and urogenital sinus.

■ NOTES

Urogenital System 13

Objectives

Be able to:

- Discuss the development of the three sets of excretory organs, with special emphasis on the development of the permanent kidneys.
- Construct and label diagrams illustrating positional changes of the kidneys during development, briefly describing congenital abnormalities of position and the renal vessels.
- Explain, with the aid of diagrams, the formation of the urinary bladder and urethra in both sexes.
- Describe the embryological basis of duplications of the superior part of the urinary tract, ectopic ureteral orifices, renal ectopia, horseshoe kidneys, congenital polycystic disease of the kidney, urachal anomalies, and exstrophy of the urinary bladder.
- Explain sex determination in human embryos and the meaning of the terms chromosomal sex, genetic sex, and phenotypic sex.
- Construct and label diagrams showing the development of (1) the ovaries and testes, (2) the genital ducts, and (3) the external genitalia.
- Discuss the embryological basis of hypospadias and ambiguous genitalia.
- Write brief notes on (1) the appearance, migration, and significance of primordial germ cells; (2) development of the seminal vesicles and prostate gland; and (3) clinically significant vestigial structures derived from the genital ducts.
- Discuss the embryological basis of intersexuality, and explain the terms true hermaphroditism and pseudohermaphroditism.
- Describe development of the suprarenal (adrenal) glands, and discuss congenital adrenocortical hyperplasia and its effects on the development of the external genitalia.
- Construct and label diagrams showing the development of the inguinal canals and descent of the testes.
- Explain the embryological basis of hydrocele and congenital inguinal hernia.

■ FIVE-CHOICE COMPLETION QUESTIONS

Directions: Directions: Each of the following statements or questions is followed by five suggested responses or completions. **Select the one best answer** in each case.

1. The human pronephros, a transitory nonfunctional "kidney," appears early in the fourth week as a few cell clusters in the _____ region of the embryo.
   A. occipital
   B. cervical
   C. thoracic
   D. abdominal
   E. pelvic

2. The human mesonephros, a transitory functional kidney, has largely degenerated by the _____ week.
   A. fifth
   B. sixth
   C. seventh
   D. eighth
   E. ninth

3. The metanephric diverticulum appears as a dorsal outgrowth from the
   A. mesonephric duct
   B. intermediate mesoderm
   C. urogenital sinus
   D. metanephric mesoderm
   E. cloaca

4. As the metanephric diverticulum grows dorsocranially, it becomes covered by _____ mesoderm
   A. splanchnic
   B. mesonephrogenic
   C. somatic
   D. metanephric
   E. intermediate

5. Incomplete division of the metanephric diverticulum (ureteric bud) results in
   A. bifid ureter
   B. supernumerary kidney
   C. duplication of the ureter
   D. partial ureteral duplication
   E. bifid ureter and supernumerary kidney

6. Embryologically, each uriniferous tubule consists of two parts, which become confluent at the junction of the
   A. renal corpuscle and the proximal convoluted tubule
   B. proximal convoluted tubule and the loop of Henle
   C. descending and ascending limbs of the loop of Henle
   D. ascending limb of the Henle loop and the distal convoluted tubule
   E. distal convoluted tubule and the collecting tubule

Five-Choice Completion Questions *Continued*

7. Exstrophy of the bladder (ectopia vesicae) often is associated with
   A. adrenal hyperplasia
   B. urachal fistula
   C. hypospadias
   D. epispadias
   E. chromosomal abnormalities

8. The metanephric diverticulum (ureteric bud) is derived from the
   A. urogenital sinus
   B. splanchnic mesoderm
   C. metanephric mesoderm
   D. somatic mesoderm
   E. mesonephric duct

9. Variations of the renal arteries are relatively common, and accessory vessels may compress the ureter, resulting in hydronephrosis and other complications. Supernumerary renal arteries are
   A. incompatible with postnatal life
   B. formed during the "descent" of the kidneys from the abdomen to the pelvis
   C. branches of the suprarenal arteries
   D. terminal or end arteries
   E. the cause of abnormal rotation of the kidneys

10. Unilateral renal agenesis was detected by ultrasonography in a near-term pregnancy that was associated with oligohydramnios. Failure of the kidney to develop probably resulted from
    A. unilateral polycystic disease
    B. degeneration of the mesonephros
    C. ureteric duplication
    D. failure of a ureteric bud to form
    E. oligohydramnios

11. With respect to hypospadias, which of the following is *false*?
    A. It occurs in about 1 of every 300 male infants.
    B. It is associated with exstrophy of the bladder.
    C. The most common types of hypospadias involve the glans penis and the body of the penis.
    D. It results from inadequate androgen production by the fetal testes or lack of adequate receptor sites for the hormones.
    E. The penile urethra is not completely fused.

12. Primordial germ cells are first recognizable early in the fourth week in the
    A. dorsal mesentery
    B. primary sex cords
    C. wall of the yolk sac
    D. gonadal ridges
    E. wall of the allantois

13. Cells of the cortical cords derived from the coelomic epithelium differentiate into
    A. follicular cells
    B. stromal cells
    C. oogonia
    D. theca folliculi
    E. primordial germ cells

Five-Choice Completion Questions *Continued*

14. The paramesonephric ducts in female embryos give rise to the
    A. paroöphoron
    B. uterine tubes
    C. inferior part of the vagina
    D. round ligament of the uterus
    E. ovarian ligament

15. The mesonephric duct in male embryos gives rise to the
    A. duct of the epoöphoron
    B. duct of Gartner
    C. ductuli efferentes
    D. ductus deferens
    E. rete testis

16. The most common cause of female pseudohermaphroditism is
    A. maternal hormone ingestion
    B. adrenocortical hyperplasia
    C. maternal arrhenoblastoma
    D. maternal progestins
    E. testicular feminization

17. Which of the following cells are derived from mesenchyme?
    A. Oogonia
    B. Interstitial cells
    C. Sertoli cells
    D. Follicular cells
    E. Spermatogonia

18. Which of the following folds give rise to labia minora?
    A. Genital
    B. Labioscrotal
    C. Urogenital
    D. Urorectal
    E. Labial

19. You are consulted about a neonate who was found to have chromatin-positive nuclei, ambiguous external genitalia, and an elevated 17-ketosteroid output. What is the most likely diagnosis?
    A. Gonadal dysgenesis with chromosomal abnormalities
    B. Female pseudohermaphroditism caused by maternal androgens
    C. Male infant with perineal hypospadias
    D. Congenital adrenocortical hyperplasia
    E. Familial male pseudohermaphroditism

20. A neonate with an apparent perineal hypospadias was found to have chromatin-negative nuclei. Gonads were palpable in the inguinal canals. The mother previously had given birth to an apparent female child with ambiguous external genitalia. This girl, now 12 years old, shows strong signs of virilization. What is the most likely diagnosis of the condition in the present infant?
    A. Female pseudohermaphroditism
    B. Perineal hypospadias
    C. Male pseudohermaphroditism
    D. Gonadal dysgenesis
    E. True hermaphroditism

Five-Choice Completion Questions *Continued*

21. The urethral groove in the female fetus usually becomes the
    - A. urethral orifice
    - B. urethra
    - C. fossa navicularis
    - D. frenulum of clitoris
    - E. vestibule of vagina

22. A 14-year-old girl was admitted because of bilateral inguinal masses. She had not begun to menstruate but showed normal breast development for her age. Her external genitalia were feminine, the vagina was shallow, but no uterus could be palpated. Her sex chromatin pattern was negative. What is the most likely diagnosis?
    - A. Male pseudohermaphroditism
    - B. Female pseudohermaphroditism
    - C. Androgen insensitivity syndrome
    - D. Inguinal hernias
    - E. Turner syndrome

23. A 16-year-old girl with a history of primary amenorrhea and cyclic pelvic pain was referred to the gynecologist. Careful examination revealed the presence of an imperforate hymen. This condition results from which of the following?
    - A. Failure of the vaginal plate to canalize
    - B. Cervical atresia
    - C. Processus vaginalis
    - D. Androgen insensitivity syndrome
    - E. Failure of the sinovaginal bulbs to develop

24. A Gartner duct cyst was diagnosed in a young patient on routine pelvic examination. This condition develops from which of the following embryonic structures?
    - A. Mesonephric duct
    - B. Mesonephric tubules
    - C. Paramesonephric duct
    - D. Urogenital folds
    - E. None of the above

25. The feminization of the external genitalia is determined by the
    - A. sinovaginal bulbs
    - B. H-Y antigen
    - C. ovaries
    - D. absence of androgens
    - E. epoöphoron

26. A bicornuate uterus was diagnosed in a 20-year-old patient who had been referred to a gynecologist on account of several miscarriages. This uterine anomaly results from
    - A. failure of fusion of the mesonephric ducts
    - B. failure of the sinovaginal bulbs to fuse
    - C. failure of fusion of the paramesonephric ducts
    - D. absence of the urogenital sinus
    - E. none of the above

Five-Choice Completion Questions *Continued*

27. A patient has been diagnosed as having a supernumerary ovary. This condition is due to
    A. absence of the paramesonephric ducts
    B. delayed migration of the primordial germ cells
    C. the testis-determining factor
    D. H-Y antigen
    E. absence of the secondary sex cords

28. The interstitial cells (of Leydig)
    A. are derived from the surface epithelium
    B. secrete müllerian-inhibiting factor
    C. influence the differentiation of the ovary
    D. produce testosterone
    E. secrete progesterone

29. An imperforate hymen was diagnosed in an infant. This structure
    A. is a mucous membrane at the entrance to the vestibule
    B. ruptures during the embryonic period
    C. separates the lumen of the vagina from the urogenital sinus in the fetus
    D. develops from the labia minora
    E. is formed by the paroöphoron

■ ANSWERS AND EXPLANATIONS

1. **B** The rudimentary pronephric "kidneys" appear in the cervical region. They have pronephric ducts that run caudally and open into the cloaca. The caudal parts of these ducts persist as the mesonephric ducts of the next set of kidneys that develop (the mesonephroi). In lower vertebrates, the pronephric ducts play an essential part in the induction of mesonephric tubules. They probably exert a similar influence in human embryos.

2. **E** The mesonephros reaches its maximum development during the embryonic period. By the beginning of the fetal period (ninth week), most of the mesonephros has degenerated, except for its duct and a few tubules, which persist as genital ducts in males or rudimentary struc-

tures in females. By the time the mesonephroi have degenerated, the metanephroi or permanent kidneys have formed and have begun to function.

3. **A** The metanephric diverticulum (ureteric bud) develops as a dorsal outgrowth from the mesonephric duct near its entry into the cloaca. The pronephric duct, which becomes the mesonephric duct, originally developed as an outgrowth from the intermediate mesoderm.

4. **D** The metanephric mass of mesoderm (metanephric blastema), derived from the nephrogenic cord, forms a mesenchymal cap over the expanded end or ampulla of the ureteric bud. This mesenchyme gives rise to the nephrons. Differentiation of

Answers and Explanations *Continued*

the nephrons is induced by an inductor substance produced by the ampulla of the ureteric bud and, later, the collecting tubules.

5. **C** Incomplete division of the metanephric diverticulum (i.e., before the renal pelvis forms) usually results in the development of two ureters. One of the ureters may have an ectopic orifice; that is, it may open into the urethra in males or the vagina in females. Complete division of the ureteric bud (before the calices form) results in incomplete ureteral duplication (i.e., bifid or Y-shaped ureter or double renal pelvis).

6. **E** The nephron, consisting of a renal corpuscle (glomerulus and Bowman capsule) and its associated tubules, develops from the metanephric mass of mesoderm around the collecting tubules. The end of a distal convoluted tubule of the nephron contacts and soon becomes confluent with a collecting tubule to form a uriniferous tubule.

7. **D** Exstrophy of the urinary bladder often is associated with epispadias, a condition in which the urethra opens on the dorsal surface of the penis. This severe anomaly is very rare. In females with epispadias, there is a fissure in the urethra that opens on the dorsal surface of the clitoris.

8. **E** The metanephric diverticulum develops as a hollow outgrowth from the mesonephric duct near its junction with the urogenital sinus. Shortly after it forms, the distal end of this outgrowth, often called the ureteric bud, expands and comes into contact with the metanephric mesoderm of the most caudal part of the nephrogenic cord.

9. **D** Supernumerary renal arteries are terminal or end arteries. If such an artery is damaged or ligated, the part of the kidney supplied by it becomes ischemic. As the kidney "ascends" from the pelvis into the abdomen, it continually acquires new branches from the aorta. Variations of the renal arteries reflect the persistence of these vessels, which normally disappear. Supernumerary renal arteries are compatible with postnatal life and play no part in the rotation of the kidneys.

10. **D** Unilateral renal agenesis arises when the ureteric bud or metanephric diverticulum on the ipsilateral side either is not formed or degenerates early. As a result, no nephrons are induced to form from the metanephric mesoderm. Whereas unilateral renal agenesis is relatively common and asymptomatic, bilateral renal agenesis is rare and fatal. The infant either is stillborn or dies almost immediately after birth.

11. **B** Hypospadias is the most common abnormality of the male external genitalia and results from incomplete fusion of the urogenital folds to form the spongy or penile urethra. It is located on the ventral surface of the penis. In severe forms of hypospadias, the penis usually is underdeveloped and curved ventrally, a condition known as chordee. Exstrophy of the bladder often is associated with epispadias, a less common defect in which the urethra opens on the dorsal surface of the penis.

12. **C** The primordial germ cells are visible early in the fourth week between the endoderm and the mesoderm of the yolk sac, near the origin of the allantois. Later during the fourth week, as the yolk sac is partially incorporated into the embryo, the primordial germ cells migrate along the dorsal mesentery of the hindgut and enter the developing gonads. They give rise to the oogonia and spermatogonia in the ovaries and the testes, respectively.

13. **A** Cells of the coelomic (germinal) epithelium give rise to cortical cords in female embryos that surround the primordial germ cells from the yolk sac. The

Answers and Explanations *Continued*

primordial germ cells become oogonia, and the coelomic epithelial cells become the follicular cells that surround the oogonia. The coelomic epithelium originally was called the germinal epithelium because it was believed to give rise to the oogonia; however, the term germinal epithelium is so firmly entrenched in the literature and in people's minds that it probably will be called by this name for some time.

14. **B** The paramesonephric ducts (formerly called müllerian ducts) give rise to the uterine tubes and uterus. Some books state that the superior four fifths of the vagina is also formed from the paramesonephric ducts, but it is believed now that the vagina is derived from the urogenital sinus and the adjacent mesenchyme.

15. **D** The mesonephric ducts (formerly called wolffian ducts) give rise to the ductus epididymidis (epididymis), ductus deferens (vas deferens), ejaculatory duct, and seminal vesicles. In females, the cranial end of the mesonephric duct may persist as a cystic appendix vesiculosa. Other parts of this duct may persist as the duct of the epoöphoron or as a Gartner duct in the broad ligament along the lateral wall of the uterus and vagina. Remnants of the duct may give rise to Gartner duct cysts.

16. **B** The usual congenital form of the adrenogenital syndrome results from an inborn error of metabolism. The pituitary gland secretes excess corticotropin, causing hyperplasia of the fetal cortex of the suprarenal glands and an overproduction of androgens. These hormones cause masculinization of female fetuses (female pseudohermaphroditism). Masculinization of fetuses by hormones administered to pregnant females or produced by maternal adrenal tumors are uncommon causes of female pseudohermaphroditism.

17. **B** The interstitial cells (of Leydig) develop from the mesenchyme located between the developing seminiferous tubules. Some cells of this embryonic connective tissue enlarge and become grouped together to form clusters of interstitial cells. These cells produce androgens during fetal life that masculinize the genital ducts and external genitalia of males. The oogonia and spermatogonia develop from primordial germ cells; the follicular and Sertoli cells develop from the primary sex cords derived from the coelomic epithelium.

18. **C** The urogenital folds in the female fetus usually do not fuse but develop into the labia minora. In the presence of androgenic substances, they may fuse. In males, the urogenital folds fuse, closing the urethral groove and forming the spongy (penile) urethra.

19. **D** An elevated 17-ketosteroid output in a chromosomal female infant with ambiguous genitalia strongly indicates congenital adrenocortical hyperplasia. These infants have an enlarged clitoris, fused labia majora, and a persistent urogenital sinus. The virilization results from an excessive production of androgens by the hyperplastic suprarenal (adrenal) glands.

20. **C** In the case presented, the apparent female infant was a male pseudohermaphrodite. Were it not for the family history of intersexuality, the most likely diagnosis would be hypospadias. Inherited defects in masculinization have been reported by many investigators. The cause of this condition is either a deficiency in the production of androgens or a defect in end-organ responsiveness to androgens.

21. **E** The urogenital folds usually do not fuse in females, and the urethral groove between them persists as the vestibule of the vagina (the space between the labia minora). The urethra and vagina open into the vestibule.

Answers and Explanations *Continued*

22. **C** The androgen insensitivity syndrome (formerly called the testicular feminization syndrome) often is considered a form of male pseudohermaphroditism, but these females do not have ambiguous external genitalia; hence, **C** is the best answer. The condition is uncommon and determined by a recessive gene. This kind of female would not pass the sex test given to females who register for the Olympics because of her chromatin-negative cells. In view of her female appearance and body structure, this is unjust.

23. **A** The vaginal plate, which is formed from the sinovaginal bulbs, gives rise to the vagina and the hymen. Imperforate hymen results from a failure of the inferior end of the vaginal plate to canalize. An imperforate hymen leads to hematocolpos, the accumulation of blood produced each month by the cyclic changes of a functional endometrium. The hymen usually presents itself on examination as a bulging, bluish membrane at the entrance to the vagina.

24. **A** Gartner duct cyst is formed from a vestigial remnant at the caudal end of the mesonephric duct. It is usually asymptomatic and is found in the wall of the vagina on routine pelvic examination. The mesonephric tubules regress in the female, leaving some rudimentary tubules, the epoöphoron and paroöphoron. The uterine tubes, uterus, and vagina are derived from the paramesonephric ducts. The labia minora develop from the urogenital folds.

25. **D** The sinovaginal bulbs give rise to the vagina. The H-Y antigen directs the formation of seminiferous tubules from the primary sex cords; its absence in the female embryo results in the development of the ovaries. Sexual differentiation of the female external genitalia results from a lack of androgens or from androgen insensitivity. The epoöphoron is a mesonephric remnant in females.

26. **C** The uterus develops from the lateral fusion of the paired paramesonephric ducts, followed by degeneration of the intervening septum. Duplication of the uterus results from a failure of this process, and it may result in two separate uteri. The mesonephric duct does not contribute to the development of the female genital tract, except for some vestigial remnants. The sinovaginal bulbs fuse and form the vaginal plate. The urinary bladder, urethra, vagina, urethral and paraurethral glands, as well as the greater vestibular glands, are derived from the urogenital sinus.

27. **B** A supernumerary ovary is an extremely rare gynecologic condition. About 20 cases have been reported in the medical literature. It results from an arrest in the migration of primordial germ cells along the dorsal mesentery of the hindgut to the genital ridges. An ectopic ovary may develop from these primordial germ cells and the surrounding mesenchyme. The paramesonephric ducts give rise to the female genital tract. The testis-determining factor influences gonadal sex differentiation; and the H-Y antigen is involved in the formation of seminiferous tubules from the primary sex cords.

28. **D** The interstitial cells (of Leydig) are derived from mesenchymal cells. By the eighth week, these cells begin to produce the androgenic hormone testosterone, which is responsible for the differentiation of the male genital ducts and external genitalia. Progesterone is secreted by the corpus luteum. Müllerian-inhibiting factor, which is produced by the sustentacular cells (of Sertoli), suppresses the development of the paramesonephric duct in the male. The development of the ovary is not influenced by the interstitial cells.

Answers and Explanations *Continued*

29. **C** The hymen is a thin fold of mucous membrane at the entrance to the vagina. It usually ruptures during the perinatal period. A condition known as imperforate hymen results when this fails to occur. The incidence of imperforate congenital hymen is about 0.1% or less. Fluid accumulation (hydrocolpos and hydrometrocolpos), especially at menarche, leads to a characteristic protruding of the membrane at the entrance to the vagina. The paraöphoron is not involved in the formation of the hymen. It is a mesonephric remnant in females.

■ FIVE-CHOICE ASSOCIATION QUESTIONS

Directions: Each group of questions below consists of a numbered list of descriptive words or phrases accompanied by a diagram with certain parts indicated by letters or by a list of lettered headings. For each numbered word or phrase, **select the lettered part or heading** that matches it correctly and then insert the letter in the space to the right of the appropriate number. Sometimes more than one numbered word or phrase may be correctly matched to the same lettered part or heading.

1. _____ Urogenital sinus
2. _____ Gives rise to collecting system of the kidney
3. _____ Partitions the cloaca
4. _____ Primordium of renal pelvis and calices
5. _____ Becomes median umbilical ligament
6. _____ Degenerates in females
7. _____ Vestigial structure in human embryos
8. _____ Temporary embryonic kidney

A. Renal agenesis
B. Nephrogenic cord
C. Metanephric diverticulum
D. Kidney lobes
E. Polycystic kidneys

9. _____ Source of nephrons
10. _____ Caused by dilations of the loops of Henle
11. _____ Oligohydramnios
12. _____ Mesonephric duct
13. _____ Intermediate mesoderm
14. _____ External evidence of them disappears during infancy

15. _____ Opens at the umbilicus
16. _____ May undergo exstrophy
17. _____ Becomes the median umbilical ligament
18. _____ Urachal sinus
19. _____ Cystic remnant of the urachus
20. _____ Short tube derived from urogenital sinus and splanchnic mesenchyme

Five-Choice Association Questions *Continued*

21. _____ Derivative of paramesonephric duct
22. _____ Corresponds to the epididymis
23. _____ Passes through the inguinal canal
24. _____ Composed of endodermal cells
25. _____ Derivative of the gubernaculum
26. _____ Derivative of the urogenital sinus
27. _____ Epoöphoron
28. _____ Gartner duct cyst

A. Adrenal hyperplasia
B. Penile hypospadias
C. Zona reticularis
D. Neuroectoderm
E. Coelomic epithelium

29. _____ Suprarenal medulla
30. _____ Gives rise to the suprarenal cortex
31. _____ Differentiates after birth
32. _____ Unfused urogenital folds
33. _____ Ambiguous external genitalia
34. _____ Associated with chordee

35. _____ Primordium of suprarenal medulla
36. _____ Gives rise to interstitial cells
37. _____ Primary sex cord
38. _____ Primordium of suprarenal cortex
39. _____ Give rise to oogonia
40. _____ Degenerates in females

A. Urogenital folds
B. Rete testis
C. Glandular plate
D. Genital tubercle
E. External oblique aponeurosis

41. _____ External spermatic fascia
42. _____ Gives rise to the clitoris
43. _____ Primary sex cords in males
44. _____ Hypospadias
45. _____ Navicular fossa
46. _____ Labia minora

■ ANSWERS AND EXPLANATIONS

1. **B** The urogenital sinus in the region indicated in the drawing gives rise to the epithelium of the urinary bladder. Distally, it also gives rise to the epithelium of the urethra, except for the terminal part of the spongy urethra (navicular fossa); this part is derived from the surface ectoderm. Other parts of the walls of these structures differentiate from the adjacent splanchnic mesenchyme.

2. **D** The metanephric diverticulum gives rise to the collecting system (i.e., the ure-

ter, renal pelvis, calices, and collecting tubules). As the diverticulum grows dorsocranially, it slowly invades the metanephric mass of mesoderm (part of the nephrogenic cord). This mesenchyme stimulates the ureteric bud to differentiate into calices and other parts of the collecting system of the permanent kidney. These structures then induce the mesenchyme to differentiate into nephrons.

3. **E** The urorectal septum is a coronal sheet or wedge of mesenchyme between

Answers and Explanations *Continued*

the allantois and the hindgut. As it grows toward the cloacal membrane, it produces infoldings of the lateral walls of the cloaca. When these infoldings fuse, they divide the cloaca into the rectum dorsally and the urogenital sinus ventrally. The urorectal septum also divides the cloacal membrane into the anal membrane and the urogenital membrane. The area of fusion of the urorectal septum with the cloacal membrane becomes the perineal body (tendinous center of the perineum).

4. **D** The metanephric diverticulum is the primordium of the renal pelvis, calices, and collecting tubules. The metanephric mesenchyme stimulates the ampulla (future renal pelvis) of the diverticulum to divide into the calices and the collecting tubules to grow into the metanephric mesenchyme from the cuplike calices. Subsequently, these tubules contact and become confluent with the nephrons to form uriniferous tubules.

5. **A** The allantois usually becomes the urachus in the fetus and forms the median umbilical ligament in the adult. Remnants of the allantois that do not become ligamentous may give rise to urachal sinuses, fistulas, or cysts. Urachal remnants are not usually detected unless they become infected.

6. **C** The mesonephros degenerates in females; almost all of it also degenerates in males. Some caudal mesonephric tubules persist in males as the efferent ductules of the testis. Before the mesonephros degenerates, the metanephric diverticulum grows from the mesonephric duct and forms the collecting system of the kidneys. Remnants of mesonephric tubules and the mesonephric duct may persist in females and give rise to cysts (e.g., cysts of the epoöphoron).

7. **A** The allantois is a vestigial structure in the human embryo; it develops during

the second week as a diverticulum from the caudal wall of the yolk sac. In some species it serves as a reservoir for excretory products, but in the human embryo it remains small and becomes the urachus (median umbilical ligament in adults). Although it may contribute to the apex of the urinary bladder, it is believed that the entire bladder develops from the urogenital sinus and the adjacent mesenchyme.

8. **C** The mesonephros is the second kidney to develop in the human embryo. The first one (pronephros) is rudimentary, but the mesonephros is believed to function for a few weeks while the metanephros or permanent kidney is developing.

9. **B** The metanephric mesenchyme in the nephrogenic cords gives rise to nephrons. When stimulated by a substance produced by the metanephric diverticulum, the metanephric mesenchyme begins to differentiate into nephrons.

10. **E** Congenital polycystic disease of the kidneys is transmitted on an autosomal basis. The cysts may result from failure of the first formed rudimentary nephrons to degenerate; later, these remnants may accumulate fluid and form cysts. Cysts may also develop from detached parts of metanephric tissue, which gives rise to rudimentary renal vesicles. It is now widely believed that these cysts are dilations of the nephrons, particularly of the loops of Henle.

11. **A** Oligohydramnios (an abnormally small volume of amniotic fluid) may be associated with renal agenesis (absence of kidneys). In the neonate, renal agenesis is suggested by large, low-set ears. This type of auricle also suggests numerical chromosomal abnormalities (e.g., trisomy 18). The fetal kidneys normally produce large amounts of urine, which is excreted into the amniotic fluid. When one or

Answers and Explanations *Continued*

both kidneys fail to form or there is urethral obstruction, the volume of amniotic fluid is small because urine production fails to occur or the urine cannot pass into the amniotic fluid.

12. **C** The metanephric diverticulum develops as an outgrowth of the mesonephric duct near its opening into the urogenital sinus. This diverticulum gives rise to the ureter, renal pelvis, calices, and collecting tubules.

13. **B** The intermediate mesoderm in the early embryo forms a longitudinal mass on each side called the nephrogenic cord. These cords give rise to nephrons, which connect with the collecting tubules formed from the ureteric buds.

14. **D** The external evidence of the kidney lobes disappears during infancy, usually by the end of the first year. Thereafter, lobes are observed only in sections of the kidney and are defined as a medullary pyramid with its cap of cortical tissue.

15. **A** A urachal sinus may open at the umbilicus and produce a discharge. The allantois, running between the umbilicus and the urinary bladder, usually becomes the urachus and, eventually, the median umbilical ligament. If the cranial part of the allantois remains patent, a sinus may form. More often, the caudal end of the allantois remains patent and gives rise to a sinus that may be continuous with the cavity of the urinary bladder.

16. **D** The posterior wall of the bladder may protrude through a defect in the anterior abdominal wall; this defect is called exstrophy of the bladder. The trigone and ureteral orifices are exposed, and urine dribbles intermittently.

17. **C** The urachus, a derivative of the allantois, usually becomes a fibrous cord after birth. Called the median umbilical liga-

ment, it extends from the apex of the urinary bladder to the umbilicus.

18. **A** Failure of closure of a portion of the intraembryonic part of the allantois may result in the formation of a urachal sinus that opens at the umbilicus or into the urinary bladder. These sinuses usually are not detected unless they become infected and produce a discharge at the umbilicus or a bladder infection.

19. **B** Remnants of the urachus that do not become fibrous and form the median umbilical ligament may accumulate fluid and become cystic. Small cysts commonly are detected in sections of the urachus or median umbilical ligament, but most cysts are not detected in living people unless they become infected and enlarge.

20. **E** The urethra in the female is a short tube that extends from the urinary bladder to an external orifice. The epithelium of the urethra is derived from the endodermal urogenital sinus; all other layers of its wall are derived from the adjacent splanchnic mesenchyme.

21. **C** The uterine tube is a derivative of the paramesonephric duct. The fused portions of these ducts give rise to the uterus.

22. **B** The epoöphoron appears in the broad ligament between the ovary and the uterine tube. It is a remnant of the mesonephric duct and some mesonephric tubules and homologous with the epididymis in males. It may become cystic and give rise to a large parovarian cyst.

23. **A** The round ligament of the uterus passes through the inguinal canal and inserts in the labium majus. It is continuous with the ovarian ligament because they are both derived from the embryonic gubernaculum.

24. **E** The vaginal plate is composed of endodermal cells derived from the urogeni-

Answers and Explanations *Continued*

tal sinus. Later, the central cells of this plate break down, forming the lumen of the vagina. Failure of this canalization to occur results in vaginal atresia.

25. **A** The round ligament is a derivative of the gubernaculum, a fibromuscular cord that passes from the inferior pole of the gonad. It descends obliquely through the developing abdominal wall (future site of the inguinal canal) and attaches to the labioscrotal fold (future labium majus).

26. **E** The vaginal plate is derived from a pair of sinovaginal bulbs that grow out from the urogenital sinus and fuse to form a solid cord of endodermal cells called the vaginal plate. The central cells of this plate subsequently degenerate, forming the lumen of the vagina.

27. **B** The epoöphoron is a vestigial structure that lies in the broad ligament between the ovary and the uterine tube. It consists of a few blind tubules connected to a short duct. If the epoöphoron becomes distended with fluid, it forms a parovarian cyst. Most are small, but some enlarge to an enormous size.

28. **D** Gartner duct cysts are derived from remnants of caudal parts of the mesonephric duct in females. They are located between the layers of the broad ligament along the lateral wall of the uterus or in the wall of the vagina. Gartner duct cysts seldom are detected unless they become infected and enlarged.

29. **D** The medulla of the suprarenal gland is derived from neuroectoderm. Neural crest cells, comparable to those that form sympathetic ganglia, invade the mesodermal suprarenal cortex on its medial side and soon become surrounded by it.

30. **E** The fetal suprarenal (adrenal) cortex is derived from mesenchymal cells that arise from the coelomic epithelium. These large cells make up most of the su-

prarenal cortex before birth, forming the massive fetal cortex. The fetal cortex gradually involutes after birth and usually is not recognizable after the first year.

31. **C** At birth, the suprarenal gland consists mainly (about 80%) of fetal cortex. The zona reticularis of the adrenal cortex forms after birth. It usually is recognizable by the end of the third year. The other two layers of the permanent cortex (zona glomerulosa and zona fasciculata) are present at birth but not fully differentiated.

32. **B** Failure of the urogenital folds to fuse in males results in hypospadias. In most cases (about 80%), the urethra opens on the ventral surface near the junction of the glans and the body (shaft) of the penis.

33. **A** Ambiguous external genitalia often indicate virilization of a female, resulting from congenital virilizing adrenal hyperplasia. Excessive production of adrenal androgens by the hyperplastic fetal cortex of the suprarenal gland causes masculinization of the external genitalia. A neonate with ambiguous genitalia, a palpable uterus, but no palpable gonads usually is a female pseudohermaphrodite whose condition is caused by adrenocortical hyperplasia.

34. **B** Chordee, a curving downward of the penis, often is associated with hypospadias, especially with the more severe types (e.g., penoscrotal hypospadias).

35. **C** The medulla of the suprarenal gland is derived from neuroectoderm. Neural crest cells, comparable to those that give rise to sympathetic nerve cells, migrate to the developing suprarenal cortex and later give rise to the suprarenal medulla.

36. **E** The mesenchyme, separating the primary sex cords, gives rise to the interstitial cells. Some cells of the mesenchyme

Answers and Explanations *Continued*

(embryonic connective tissue) enlarge and become grouped together. They produce androgens during the fetal period that stimulate development of the mesonephric ducts and inhibit development of the paramesonephric ducts. These sex hormones also cause masculinization of the external genitalia.

37. **A** The primary sex cords give rise to the seminiferous tubules, tubuli recti, and rete testis. They lose their connections with the surface epithelium as the tunica albuginea forms.

38. **D** The suprarenal cortex, derived from mesoderm, is first recognizable as a mass of mesenchymal cells on each side between the root of the mesentery and the developing gonad. Before birth, most of the suprarenal cortex (about 80%) consists of fetal cortex. This zone rapidly involutes after birth, losing about half its mass in 2 weeks.

39. **B** The primordial germ cells are the precursors of oogonia in female embryos and spermatogonia in male embryos. The primordial germ cells come from the yolk sac to the gonads and soon become incorporated into the primary sex cords.

40. **A** The primary sex cords normally degenerate in female embryos, but during the fetal period, secondary sex cords (called cortical cords) extend from the surface epithelium into the underlying mesenchyme. Primordial germ cells are incorporated into the cortical cords and give rise to the oogonia. The follicular cells that surround the oogonia are derived from the cortical cords.

41. **E** The external spermatic fascia is an extension of the external oblique aponeurosis. As the testis and its associated structures descend, they become ensheathed by fascial extensions of the abdominal wall. These extensions are produced by the processus vaginalis as it projects through the abdominal wall along the path formed by the gubernaculum.

42. **D** The genital tubercle elongates in both sexes to form a phallus. In females, growth of the phallus normally slows after the eighth week; it becomes the relatively small clitoris. In the presence of androgenic substances (e.g., administered to the mother or produced by hyperplastic fetal suprarenal glands), the clitoris elongates to form a penis-like structure and the labia majora fuse.

43. **B** The primary sex cords in male embryos condense and extend into the medulla of the developing testis. Here they branch, and their ends anastomose to form the rete testis.

44. **A** Hypospadias is a common abnormal condition of the urethra (about 1 in 300 males) resulting from failure of fusion of the urogenital folds. In some cases, the labioscrotal folds also fail to fuse and result in severe forms of hypospadias (e.g., penoscrotal and perineal hypospadias). This arrest of development is the result of an inadequate production of androgens by the fetal testes.

45. **C** The terminal portion of the penile urethra, the navicular fossa, is derived from the glandular plate. This plate is formed by an ectodermal ingrowth into the glans penis from the surface epithelium. Subsequent splitting of this plate forms a groove on the ventral surface of the glans. Closure of the urethral groove moves the external urethral orifice to the tip of the glans penis and joins this part of the spongy urethra with that formed by fusion of the urogenital folds.

46. **A** The labia minora develop from the urogenital folds. In male embryos that receive adequate amounts of androgenic hormones, the urogenital folds fuse to form the spongy urethra.

Cardiovascular System 14

Objectives

Be able to:

- Illustrate with simple, labeled sketches the events that occur between the third and sixth weeks that change the primordial heart tube into the shape that characterizes the adult heart.
- Explain partitioning of the primordial atrium and ventricle, discussing clinically significant atrial and ventricular septal defects.
- Construct and label diagrams illustrating the course of the fetal circulation and the changes that normally occur at birth and during the postnatal period.
- Summarize the major events in the transformation of the embryonic aortic arch system into the adult arterial pattern.
- Discuss the relatively common aortic arch anomalies (especially patent ductus arteriosus and coarctation of the aorta).
- Outline the embryological basis of the following congenital anomalies: double aortic arch, right aortic arch, and retroesophageal subclavian artery.

■ FIVE-CHOICE COMPLETION QUESTIONS

Directions: Each of the following statements or questions is followed by five suggested responses or completions. **Select the one best answer** in each case.

1. Incomplete fusion of the endocardial cushions usually is associated with which of the following types of atrial septal defect (ASD)?
   A. Secundum-type ASD
   B. Primum-type ASD
   C. Common atrium
   D. Probe patent ASD
   E. Sinus venosus–type ASD

2. The fetal left atrium is mainly derived from the
   A. primordial pulmonary vein
   B. right pulmonary vein
   C. primitive atrium
   D. sinus venarum
   E. sinus venosus

3. Congenital heart disease is the most common cardiac condition in childhood and most frequently results from
   A. maternal medications
   B. mutant genes
   C. rubella virus
   D. fetal distress
   E. genetic and environmental factors

Five-Choice Completion Questions *Continued*

4. The most common type of defect of the cardiac septa is
    A. secundum-type ASD
    B. muscular-type ventricular septal defect (VSD)
    C. primum-type ASD
    D. membranous-type VSD
    E. sinus venosus-type ASD

5. Closure of the foramen primum results from fusion of the
    A. septum primum and the septum secundum
    B. septum secundum and the septum spurium
    C. septum primum and the endocardial cushions
    D. septum secundum and the endocardial cushions
    E. septum primum and the right sinoatrial valve

6. The fetal right atrium is mainly derived from the
    A. primordial pulmonary vein   D. sinus venarum
    B. right pulmonary vein   E. sinus venosus
    C. primordial atrium

7. The most common congenital anomaly of the heart and great vessels associated with the congenital rubella syndrome is
    A. coarctation of the aorta   D. ASD
    B. tetralogy of Fallot   E. VSD
    C. patent ductus arteriosus

8. The cardiovascular system reaches a functional state at the end of the _____ week.
    A. second   D. fifth
    B. third   E. sixth
    C. fourth

9. A female infant with congestive heart failure and continuous systolic and diastolic murmurs was diagnosed as having a patent ductus arteriosus. Which of the following statements is correct?
    A. The ductus arteriosus is a remnant of the left fourth aortic arch.
    B. The ductus arteriosus is closed during fetal development.
    C. The ductus arteriosus shunts blood from the umbilical vein to the inferior vena cava.
    D. The ductus arteriosus closes just before birth.
    E. In the fetus, most of the blood from the pulmonary trunk flows into the aorta.

Five-Choice Completion Questions *Continued*

10. On routine examination of an infant who has failed to thrive and has poor weight, a loud murmur was detected at the lower left sternal border. A diagnosis of VSD was made, and subsequently, the absence of the membranous part of the atrioventricular septum was confirmed by two-dimensional echocardiography. Membranous VSD _____.
    A. arises from failure of subendocardial tissue of endocardial cushions to fuse with the aorticopulmonary septum and muscular part of the interventricular septum
    B. results from excessive resorption of myocardial tissue
    C. causes shunting of blood from the right ventricle into the left ventricle
    D. is found only in association with an ASD
    E. is a rare condition and the less common type of VSD

11. Transposition of the great arteries was diagnosed in a male infant with obvious cyanosis and mild tachypnea. This condition results from which of the following?
    A. Abnormal resorption of the septum primum
    B. Failure of the endocardial cushions to fuse
    C. Faulty partitioning of the bulbus cordis and truncus arteriosus
    D. Involution of the ductus arteriosus
    E. Abnormal transformation of the sixth aortic arches

12. A secundum ASD was detected in a young child. Regarding this congenital anomaly, which of the following is *incorrect?*
    A. It occurs more frequently in males than in females.
    B. It is located in the area of the fossa ovalis.
    C. It is usually asymptomatic during childhood.
    D. It results from abnormal resorption of the septum primum.
    E. It includes defects of the septum primum and septum secundum.

■ ANSWERS AND EXPLANATIONS

1. **B** The primum-type ASD associated with an endocardial cushion defect is the second most common type of clinically significant ASD. The incomplete form of endocardial cushion defect is relatively common, in which the septum primum does not fuse with the endocardial cushions. As a result, there is a patent foramen primum and often a cleft in the anterior (or septal) leaflet of the mitral valve.

2. **A** Most of the wall of the left atrium is smooth and derived by absorption of the primordial pulmonary vein. At first, the common pulmonary vein opens into the primordial left atrium, but as the atrium expands, portions of this vein are incorporated into the wall of the atrium. The primordial atrium forms only a relatively small part of the adult left atrium (i.e., the left auricle).

3. **E** Congenital heart disease usually is not caused by a single factor. Heart anomalies are found in single-gene disorders, but most fit the criteria for multifactorial inheritance. Rubella virus is an agent known to be associated with patent ductus arteriosus and pulmonary stenosis. Maternal medications (e.g., thalidomide) rarely are associated with congenital heart disease; however, most heart defects result from unknown causes, probably a complex interaction of genetic and environmental factors.

Answers and Explanations *Continued*

4. **D** Membranous-type VSD is the most common type of heart defect. This anomaly usually results from failure of the membranous portion of the interventricular septum to form at the end of the seventh week.

5. **C** As the septum primum grows toward the fusing endocardial cushions, the foramen primum becomes progressively smaller. The septum primum eventually fuses with the left side of the fused endocardial cushions and obliterates the foramen primum.

6. **E** Most of the wall of the right atrium is smooth and derived by absorption of the right horn of the sinus venosus. The sinus venosus initially opens into the right atrium, but as the atrium expands, the right horn of the sinus venosus gradually is incorporated into the right atrium and becomes the smooth-walled part, called the sinus venarum. The primordial atrium is represented by the right auricle, a small, muscular pouch. The smooth part (sinus venarum) and the rough part (auricle) are demarcated internally by a vertical ridge, the crista terminalis, and externally by a shallow inconspicuous groove, the sulcus terminalis.

7. **C** The most frequent anomalies associated with the congenital rubella syndrome are congenital heart disease (especially patent ductus arteriosus and pulmonary stenosis), deafness, and blindness (cataract). These anomalies result from maternal infection during the first trimester of pregnancy. Rubella infection during the second trimester can cause deafness, microcephaly, and mental retardation. The influence of teratogens such as rubella on development of the heart and great vessels is well known, but the role of other viral infections and drugs is inconclusive.

8. **B** Cardiovascular development is first evident in the cardiogenic area at about 18 days. By the end of the third week, embryonic and extraembryonic vessels are connected to the heart and a slow circulation of blood has begun. When the heart begins to beat about a day later, the circulation becomes an ebb and flow type.

9. **E** The ductus arteriosus is derived from the left sixth aortic arch; the left fourth aortic arch contributes to the formation of the arch of the aorta. In the fetus, the lumen of the ductus arteriosus is large and permits the flow of blood from the pulmonary trunk into the aorta. Pulmonary blood flow in the fetus is low because of the high pulmonary resistance. The ductus arteriosus constricts at birth and usually is functionally closed 10 to 15 hours later. With involution, it becomes the ligamentum arteriosum. A patent ductus arteriosus is more commonly found in females than in males. With only few exceptions, all patients with patent ductus arteriosus should have medical or surgical closure.

10. **A** VSD is the most common type of cardiac defect, and a defect in the membranous part of the septum is the most common type of VSD. It is caused by a failure of the subendocardial tissues of the fused endocardial cushions to fuse with both the aorticopulmonary septum and the muscular part of the interventricular septum. VSDs are embryologically unrelated to ASDs. A VSD causes shunting of left ventricular blood into the right ventricle. Spontaneous closure of VSDs during the first few months after birth is relatively common, but in other cases, medical management or surgery is indicated to deal with the accompanying congestive heart failure.

11. **C** It is believed that failure of the aorticopulmonary septum to pursue a spiral course during the division of the bulbus cordis and the truncus arteriosus results in the aorta arising from the right ventri-

Answers and Explanations *Continued*

cle and the pulmonary trunk from the left ventricle. This is one of the most common cardiac defects seen in infancy, predominantly in males. Other congenital cardiac anomalies may be present in neonates with transposition of the great vessels.

12. **A** Secundum ASDs (ostium secundum defects) occur more frequently in females than in males (3:1). The lesions are lo-

cated in the area of the fossa ovalis and involve both the septum primum and septum secundum. Children with ASDs are usually asymptomatic, and only later symptoms may appear. Abnormal resorption of the septum primum during formation of the septum secundum, excessive resorption of the septum primum, or defective development of the septum secundum provides an embryological explanation for secundum ASDs.

■ FIVE-CHOICE ASSOCIATION QUESTIONS

Directions: Each group of questions below consists of a numbered list of descriptive words or phrases accompanied by a diagram with certain parts indicated by letters or by a list of lettered headings. For each numbered word or phrase, **select the lettered part or heading** that matches it correctly, and then insert the letter in the space to the right of the appropriate number. Sometimes more than one numbered word or phrase may be correctly matched to the same lettered part or heading.

1. _____ Directs blood into the left atrium
2. _____ Carries relatively little blood
3. _____ Remains of the septum primum
4. _____ Opening in the septum secundum
5. _____ Carries well-oxygenated blood
6. _____ Septum secundum

A. Ductus arteriosus
B. Septum primum
C. Right sixth aortic arch
D. Sinus venosus
E. Umbilical vein

7. _____ Ligamentum teres
8. _____ Carries poorly oxygenated blood into the right atrium
9. _____ Arterial shunt
10. _____ Floor of the fossa ovalis
11. _____ Ductus venosus
12. _____ Right recurrent laryngeal nerve

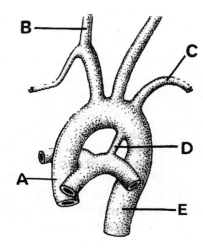

A. Coarctation
B. Infundibular stenosis
C. Patent ductus arteriosus
D. VSD
E. Tetralogy of Fallot

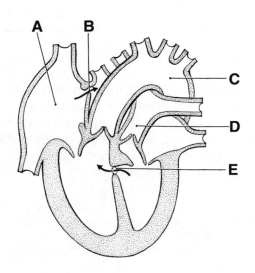

13. _____ Derivative of an intersegmental artery
14. _____ Forms from the sixth aortic arch artery
15. _____ Derived from the truncus arteriosus
16. _____ Formed by fusion of the dorsal aortae
17. _____ Derived from the third aortic arch artery
18. _____ Becomes ligamentous during infancy

19. _____ Pulmonary valve stenosis
20. _____ Rubella syndrome
21. _____ Right ventricular hypertrophy
22. _____ Most common cardiac defect
23. _____ Constriction of aorta
24. _____ Overriding aorta

25. _____ A defect in the area of the fossa ovalis
26. _____ Normally communicates with the right ventricle
27. _____ Closes by the end of the seventh week
28. _____ Is formed from the dorsal aorta
29. _____ Is partly derived from the sinus venosus

■ ANSWERS AND EXPLANATIONS

1. **C** Blood from the inferior vena cava is directed by the inferior border of the septum secundum (crista dividens) through the foramen ovale into the left atrium.

2. **D** The pulmonary veins carry relatively little blood to the left atrium before birth because the lungs are not functioning. When the lungs expand at birth and the pulmonary vascular resistance falls, there is a marked increase in pulmonary blood flow with a consequent increased flow to the left atrium through the pulmonary veins.

3. **E** The remains of the septum primum are represented here by the valve of the foramen ovale. This valve is forced open by blood from the inferior vena cava that is directed through the foramen ovale by the crista dividens (inferior edge of septum secundum). The foramen ovale normally closes at birth when pressure in the left atrium rises above that in the right atrium.

4. **B** The foramen ovale is a normal opening in the septum secundum. It permits well-oxygenated blood from the placenta that comes from the inferior vena cava to enter the left atrium. If the foramen ovale fails to close at birth, a cardiac anomaly known as secundum-type ASD exists. This common congenital heart defect accounts for about 8% of cases of congenital heart disease.

5. **A** The inferior vena cava carries well-oxygenated blood from the placenta. This fetal blood returns from the placenta in the umbilical vein. About half the blood passes through the hepatic sinusoids before entering the inferior vena cava. The other half is shunted by way of the ductus venosus directly from the umbilical vein to the inferior vena cava.

6. **C** The septum secundum is the second part of the interatrial septum to form.

The crista dividens, its inferior border, is indicated by the pointer. It directs most of the blood from the inferior vena cava through the opening in the septum secundum (foramen ovale) into the left atrium. The smaller portion of blood, turned back by the septum secundum, enters the right ventricle.

7. **E** The intra-abdominal portion of the fetal umbilical vein becomes the adult ligamentum teres and passes from the umbilicus to the porta hepatis, where it attaches to the left branch of the portal vein.

8. **D** The sinus venosus initially is a separate chamber of the heart that opens into the caudal wall of the right atrium. The right horn of the sinus venosus becomes incorporated into the wall of the right atrium and forms the smooth-walled portion called the sinus venarum. The left horn of the sinus venosus becomes the coronary sinus.

9. **A** The ductus arteriosus is an arterial shunt that carries blood from the left pulmonary artery to the arch of the aorta before birth. Because the lungs are not functioning, most of the blood in the pulmonary artery bypasses the lungs and enters the descending aorta.

10. **B** The floor of the fossa ovalis in the interatrial septum is formed by tissue derived from the septum primum (valve of the foramen ovale). When the pressure in the left atrium rises at birth, the valve of the foramen ovale closes and later fuses with the septum secundum. This valvular tissue forms the floor of the fossa ovalis.

11. **E** About half the blood coming from the placenta in the umbilical vein is shunted through the liver by way of the ductus venosus into the inferior vena cava. The remainder of the blood enters the liver and is carried to the inferior vena cava by the hepatic veins.

Answers and Explanations *Continued*

12. **C** The recurrent laryngeal nerves hook around the sixth pair of aortic arch arteries. On the right, the distal part of the sixth arch artery and the fifth aortic arch artery degenerate, leaving the right recurrent laryngeal nerve hooked around the right subclavian artery. On the left, the recurrent laryngeal nerve hooks around the ductus arteriosus (ligamentum arteriosum in the adult) and the arch of the aorta.

13. **C** The left subclavian artery, unlike the right subclavian artery, is not derived from an aortic arch artery or the dorsal aorta. It develops from the seventh intersegmental artery that arises from the descending aorta and moves cranially as the arch of the aorta forms.

14. **D** The ductus arteriosus develops from the distal portion of the left sixth aortic arch artery. It passes from the left pulmonary artery to the aorta and, before birth, carries most of the blood from the pulmonary trunk into the aorta. The lungs are not functioning and so require little blood. The ductus arteriosus usually constricts slightly after birth and closes anatomically during the first 3 months.

15. **A** The proximal part of the ascending aorta is derived from the truncus arteriosus when it is divided by the aorticopulmonary septum. The remainder of the ascending aorta develops from the aortic sac.

16. **E** The descending aorta forms when the paired dorsal aortae of the embryo fuse just caudal to the heart. The cranial portion of the right dorsal aorta normally involutes, but if it persists, a double aortic arch forms that may compress the trachea and esophagus.

17. **B** The right common carotid artery is derived from the proximal part of the right third aortic arch artery. This artery also gives rise to the internal carotid artery on this side.

18. **D** The ductus arteriosus constricts slightly at birth but usually is patent for a week or so. Proliferation of endothelial and fibrous tissues of the ductus arteriosus usually results in its anatomic closure by the end of the third month.

19. **E** Stenosis of the pulmonary tract is one of the four anomalies of the heart and great vessels included in the tetralogy of Fallot. These severe defects are regarded as the most important of the cardiac defects that produce cyanosis.

20. **C** Patent ductus arteriosus is the most common congenital anomaly of the heart and great vessels associated with maternal rubella infection during the first trimester.

21. **B** Enlargement and hypertrophy of the right ventricle result from high blood pressure, often resulting from pulmonary stenosis. The narrowing may occur at the infundibulum of the right ventricle, the pulmonary valve, or, less commonly, in the pulmonary trunk. **E** is also correct, but **B** is the better answer.

22. **D** VSD is the most common cardiac defect, accounting for about 22% of cases of congenital heart disease. It may occur with various other cardiac defects (e.g., in tetralogy of Fallot). VSD most commonly consists of an opening (1 to 15 mm in diameter) in the membranous portion of the interventricular septum.

23. **A** In preductal coarctation, the aorta constricts superior to the ductus arteriosus, which usually is patent. More often, the constriction is inferior to the ductus (postductal coarctation).

24. **E** Overriding aorta or an aorta arising directly over a VSD, and thus overriding both ventricular cavities, is an essential feature of the tetralogy of Fallot. People with this group of cardiac abnormalities are cyanotic because not enough blood

Answers and Explanations *Continued*

flows to the lungs for oxygenation. As long as the ductus arteriosus remains patent, there is compensatory flow through it from the aorta to the pulmonary arteries. If the ductus closes, as commonly occurs, the deficit in pulmonary circulation increases.

25. **B**   Atrial septal defect is a common congenital anomaly. It occurs more frequently in females than in males. A patent foramen ovale is the most common form of ASD, resulting from incomplete fusion between the septum secundum and the flap-type valve of the foramen ovale. Before birth, most of the blood entering the right atrium is shunted through the foramen ovale into the left atrium. After birth, the pressure in the left atrium rises with the return of blood from the lungs. As a result, the septum primum becomes pressed against the septum secundum, and eventually the foramen ovale is permanently closed. Of the main types of ASD, the secundum ASD is most common and is located in the area of the fossa ovalis.

26. **D**   The pulmonary trunk normally communicates with the right ventricle, transporting deoxygenated blood to the lungs after birth. In typical cases of transposition of the great arteries, the aorta arises from the right ventricle anteriorly, and on the left the pulmonary artery arises from the left ventricle posteriorly. Transposition of the great arteries is the most common cause of cyanotic heart disease in newborn infants, and it is often found in association with other cardiac anomalies. According to the conal growth hypothesis, the aorticopulmonary septum fails to pursue a spiral course during partitioning of the bulbus cordis and truncus aorticus.

27. **E**   A crescentic interventricular foramen, between the free edge of the muscular part of the interventricular septum and the fused endocardial cushions, permits blood to pass between the right and left ventricles until the seventh week. With the formation of the membranous part of the interventricular septum by the end of the seventh week, the interventricular foramen is obliterated. The membranous part of the interventricular septum, derived from the fused endocardial cushions, merges with the bulbar ridges of the aorticopulmonary septum and the muscular part of the interventricular septum.

28. **C**   The distal part of the arch of the aorta is derived from the left dorsal aorta; its proximal part is formed from the fourth aortic arch and the aortic sac. In this case of transposition of the great arteries, the aorta is shown arising from the right ventricle. Coarctation (constriction) of the aorta almost invariably is located where the ductus arteriosus connects with the aortic arch and the descending aorta.

29. **A**   The formation and subsequent fusion of the septum primum and septum secundum divide the primordial atrium into a right atrium and a left atrium. Initially, the sinus venosus opens into the dorsal wall of the primordial right atrium. By the end of the fourth week, the right horn of the sinus venosus is larger than the left. The right horn of the sinus venosus becomes incorporated into the wall of the right atrium, and the left horn forms the coronary sinus. The smooth part of the wall of the right atrium is known as the sinus venarum because it is derived from the sinus venosus.

Skeletal and Muscular Systems

Objectives

Be able to:

- Construct and label diagrams showing the development and early differentiation of somites.
- Discuss briefly the histogenesis of skeletal, cardiac, and smooth muscle.
- Describe endochondral and intramembranous bone formation.
- Construct and label diagrams showing the development of the different types of joint.
- Describe the development of a typical vertebra.
- Make and label simple sketches of the fetal skull showing the bones, fontanelles, and sutures.
- Discuss briefly achondroplasia, spina bifida occulta, cervical and lumbar ribs, acrania, and craniosynostosis.

■ FIVE-CHOICE COMPLETION QUESTIONS

Directions: Each of the following statements or questions is followed by five suggested responses or completions. **Select the one best answer** in each case.

1. Which of the following bones is *not* mainly formed by endochondral ossification?
   A. Humerus
   B. Mandible
   C. Hyoid
   D. Occipital
   E. Tibia

2. Which of the following bones is completely formed by intramembranous ossification?
   A. Stapes
   B. Parietal
   C. Clavicle
   D. Radius
   E. Sphenoid

3. The most common type of accessory rib is a _____ rib.
   A. lumbar
   B. forked
   C. cervical
   D. thoracic
   E. fused

4. Myoblasts from the occipital myotomes are believed to give rise to the muscles of the
   A. eye
   B. ear
   C. neck
   D. tongue
   E. pharynx

Five-Choice Completion Questions *Continued*

5. The pharyngeal and laryngeal muscles develop from mesenchyme derived from the
   A. preotic myotomes
   B. occipital myotomes
   C. splanchnic mesoderm
   D. somatic mesoderm
   E. pharyngeal arches

6. Which of the following bones is *not* derived mainly from the cartilaginous viscerocranium?
   A. Malleus
   B. Incus
   C. Stapes
   D. Occipital
   E. Hyoid

7. Increase in the size of the calvaria (brain case) is greatest during the first _____ years.
   A. 2
   B. 3
   C. 5
   D. 7
   E. 9

8. The neonate's face is relatively small compared with the calvaria. Enlargement of the facial region during childhood mainly results from an increase in the size of the
   A. paranasal sinuses
   B. deciduous teeth
   C. nose and jaws
   D. permanent teeth
   E. brain and calvaria

9. The skeleton shows clearly on radiographs (x-ray films) by the beginning of the _____ week.
   A. 7th
   B. 9th
   C. 11th
   D. 13th
   E. 15th

10. Achondroplasia was diagnosed in a child. With respect to this disorder, all the following are correct *except*:
    A. Most common cause of dwarfism
    B. Autosomal recessive disorder
    C. Autosomal dominant disorder
    D. Limbs are short
    E. Ossification at the epiphyseal cartilage plates is disturbed

11. Congenital torticollis was diagnosed in an infant whose head was tilted to the right with the chin turned to the left. Which of the following is involved?
    A. Right sternocleidomastoid muscle
    B. Left sternocleidomastoid muscle
    C. Fusion of the cervical vertebrae
    D. Vertebral anomalies
    E. Absence of right pectoralis major muscle

■ ANSWERS AND EXPLANATIONS

1. **B** The mandible forms almost entirely by intramembranous ossification. Some endochondral ossification occurs in a small portion of the anterior part of the mandible and at its condyle. The mesenchyme in the mandibular process of the first pharyngeal arch condenses around the first arch cartilage (Meckel cartilage) to form a dense fibromembranous tissue; this undergoes intramembranous ossification as the cartilage degenerates. Hence, endochondral ossification does not occur in the Meckel cartilage, as one might expect.

2. **B** The parietal and other flat bones of the neurocranium develop by intramembranous ossification. The clavicle begins to develop by intramembranous ossification, but later develops growth cartilages at each end that give rise to most of the bone.

3. **A** Lumbar ribs are the most common type of accessory rib, but they usually are of no clinical significance. Cervical ribs are attached to the seventh cervical vertebra. They may be unilateral or bilateral, complete or incomplete. A cervical rib usually causes no symptoms; however, the subclavian artery and the inferior part of the brachial plexus may cross over the cervical rib. In these cases, the rib may exert pressure on these structures and give rise to pain and/or muscular atrophy in the upper limb.

4. **D** There initially are four occipital somites and, hence, four occipital myotomes. The first pair of somites disappears, and the myotomes of the others give rise to mesenchyme that forms the tongue muscles. When the myoblasts that give rise to these muscles migrate to the tongue, they carry their nerve supply with them.

5. **E** The mesenchyme that gives rise to the myoblasts that form the pharyngeal and laryngeal muscles is derived from the fourth and sixth pharyngeal arches. These muscles are innervated by the vagus nerve (CN X), the nerve that supplies these arches.

6. **D** The occipital bone is derived mainly by ossification of the dorsal part of the cartilaginous neurocranium. The portion of this bone superior to the highest nuchal line develops by intramembranous ossification. The cartilaginous viscerocranium consists of the cartilaginous skeleton of the first two pairs of pharyngeal arches. Parts of the cartilages in these arches undergo endochondral ossification to form bone (e.g., the styloid process of the temporal bone).

7. **A** Growth of the calvaria is rapid during infancy, especially during the first 2 years. This growth is related primarily to the extensive development of the brain during this period. The calvaria normally increases slightly in capacity until 15 or 16 years of age.

8. **A** Enlargement of the frontal and facial regions of the postnatal skull results mainly from the increase in size of the paranasal sinuses. These air sinuses develop during the late fetal period and infancy as small diverticula of the lateral walls of the nasal cavities. During childhood, these sinuses also extend into the maxilla, ethmoid, frontal, and sphenoid bones. This causes enlargement of the face. There is concurrent development of the jaws as the teeth develop and erupt.

9. **E** Although the fetal skeleton may be visualized earlier than 15 weeks on radiographs, it usually is not clearly displayed until after the 14th week. X-ray investigations often raise concerns about the hazards of ionizing radiation. Embryos are particularly radiosensitive during the period of organogenesis. The fetal gonads and the brain are radiosensitive throughout the fetal period. Because of this, ultrasound scans of the uterus often are used

Answers and Explanations *Continued*

to diagnose twins, locate the placenta, and study the fetal skull. There is no increased incidence of congenital abnormalities or evidence of tissue damage caused by sound energy in infants of mothers who have undergone sonography.

10. **B** Achondroplasia is an autosomal dominant disorder. It is the most common cause of dwarfism and occurs with a frequency of about 1 in 10,000 births. The limbs are short, the head is relatively large, and there is thoracic kyphosis with protrusion of the abdomen. Disturbance of endochondral ossification at the epi-physeal cartilage plates results in the short limbs.

11. **A** The right sternocleidomastoid muscle is shortened, resulting in the ear being closer to the shoulder on the affected side and the chin rotated toward the opposite side. The cause is not known. Because torticollis has been observed in infants delivered by cesarean section, it has been suggested that factors other than birth trauma may be involved. Absence of the sternal part of the pectoralis major muscle is not uncommon, but it is unrelated to congenital torticollis.

■ FIVE-CHOICE ASSOCIATION QUESTIONS

Directions: Each group of questions below consists of a numbered list of descriptive words or phrases accompanied by a diagram with certain parts indicated by letters or by a list of lettered headings. For each numbered word or phrase, **select the lettered part or heading** that matches it correctly and then insert the letter in the space to the right of the appropriate number. Sometimes more than one numbered word or phrase may be correctly matched to the same lettered part or heading.

A. Centrum
B. Epiphyseal plates
C. Frontal bone
D. Anterior fontanelle
E. Cartilaginous viscerocranium

1. _____ Closes during the second year
2. _____ Forms by intramembranous ossification
3. _____ Partly within the first and second pharyngeal arches
4. _____ Growth of long bones
5. _____ Primary ossification center
6. _____ Styloid process

7. _____ Associated with the first pharyngeal arch cartilage
8. _____ Part of the cartilaginous viscerocranium
9. _____ Forms in the maxillary prominence of the first pharyngeal arch
10. _____ Part of the cartilaginous neurocranium
11. _____ Forms in the mandibular prominence of the first pharyngeal arch
12. _____ Part of the membranous neurocranium

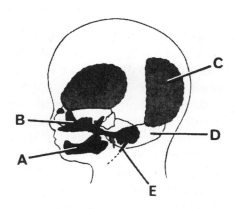

Five-Choice Completion Questions *Continued*

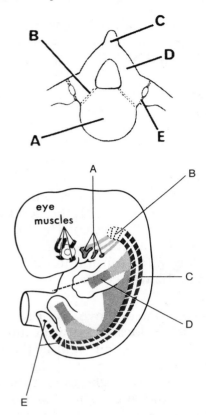

13. _____ Articulates with the centrum
14. _____ Neurocentral joint
15. _____ Replaced by a synovial joint
16. _____ Centrum
17. _____ Its cartilage is ossified during infancy
18. _____ Disappears during childhood

19. _____ Form the tongue muscles
20. _____ Normally regress in the embryo
21. _____ Form the scalene muscles
22. _____ Give rise to the muscles of mastication
23. _____ Muscles originate from somites

■ ANSWERS AND EXPLANATIONS

1. **D** The anterior fontanelle, located where the two parietal bones and the halves of the frontal bone meet, usually closes about the middle of the second year. Palpation of this fontanelle during infancy gives information about ossification of the skull and intracranial pressure.

2. **C** The frontal bone, part of the membranous neurocranium, develops by intramembranous ossification from two primary centers. The halves of the frontal bone begin to fuse during the second year, and the frontal or metopic suture usually is obliterated by the eighth year.

3. **E** The ends of the cartilaginous rods in the first and second pairs of pharyngeal arches reach the ventral surface of the neurocranium in the region of the devel-

oping ears. Later, they undergo endochondral ossification to form the lesser cornua and the superior part of the body of the hyoid bone.

4. **B** During the later stages of postnatal bone growth, the mass of cartilage between the diaphysis and epiphysis decreases in thickness to form a comparatively thin cartilage, the epiphyseal cartilage plate. This plate is of importance for growth of long bones. At the termination of growth in the bone, the epiphyseal plate disappears and the epiphysis unites with the diaphysis.

5. **A** Most of the body of a typical vertebra (thoracic and lumbar) is ossified from a primary center, the centrum, which appears during the eighth week. At birth,

Answers and Explanations *Continued*

the bone of the centrum is separated from the separate halves of the vertebral arch of cartilage by the neurocentral joints.

6. **E** The styloid process of the temporal bone develops by endochondral ossification of part of the dorsal end of the cartilage of the second pharyngeal arch (Reichert cartilage). The cartilages of the first two pairs of pharyngeal arches constitute the cartilaginous viscerocranium.

7. **A** Development of the mandible is associated with Meckel cartilage, the cartilage in the mandibular prominence of the first pharyngeal arch. As this cartilage degenerates, the condensed mesenchyme near it undergoes intramembranous ossification to form the mandible (bone of lower jaw).

8. **E** The styloid process of the temporal bone and the malleus, incus, and stapes are derived from the cartilaginous viscerocranium (skeleton of the embryonic jaws).

9. **B** The maxilla forms in the maxillary prominence of the first pharyngeal arch by intramembranous ossification. It is part of the membranous viscerocranium, as are the mandible, zygomatic, and squamous temporal bones.

10. **D** The occipital bone ossifies partly by endochondral ossification of the posterior part of the cartilaginous neurocranium. This plate of cartilage forms in the base of the developing skull by the fusion of several paired cartilages.

11. **A** The mandible is the part of the membranous viscerocranium that develops mainly by intramembranous ossification around the degenerating cartilage of the first pharyngeal arch.

12. **C** The parietal and other flat bones of the skull are parts of the membranous

neurocranium that develop by intramembranous ossification. At birth, they are separated by connective tissue sutures.

13. **D** Each half of the vertebral arch, called a lamina, is ossified from a primary ossification center. At birth, the halves of the arch are separated from each other dorsally by cartilage and from the centrum by the cartilaginous neurocentral joints. These joints disappear when the vertebral arch fuses with the centrum (usually about the fifth year). The halves of the vertebral arch fuse during the first year; failure of this fusion to occur results in spina bifida occulta.

14. **B** As stated above, the neurocentral joints are located between the centrum and the vertebral arch. In the superior cervical vertebrae, the centra unite with the vertebral arches about the third year, but in the inferior lumbar vertebrae, union is not completed until the sixth year.

15. **E** The ribs are connected to the costal processes of thoracic vertebrae at costovertebral joints. As the ribs and vertebrae ossify, joints develop between the tubercles of the ribs and the transverse processes of the vertebrae.

16. **A** The major portion of the body of a typical vertebra is formed by the centrum. It is ossified from a primary center that appears dorsal to the notochord. The centrum occasionally is ossified from bilateral primary centers.

17. **C** The vertebrae form by the ossification of cartilaginous bone models. Primary centers appear during the early fetal period—one in each half of the vertebral arch and one in the centrum. At birth, the ossified halves of the vertebral arch are still separated from each other by cartilage **(C).** This cartilage is ossified during the first year.

Answers and Explanations *Continued*

18. **B** The vertebral arch (neural arch) during infancy and early childhood is separated from the bone of the centrum by persistent bilateral zones of cartilage (neurocentral joints). These two lateral zones are ossified during the fifth or sixth year.

19. **B** The first pair of four occipital myotomes degenerate. Myoblasts from the remaining three myotomes migrate from the occipital region to the floor of the pharynx and form the striated muscles of the tongue, with the exception of the palatoglossus muscle. The hypoglossal nerve (CN XII) supplies all the muscles of the tongue except for the palatoglossus muscle, which is supplied by the pharyngeal branch of the vagus nerve (CN X).

20. **E** The paired cuboidal somites begin to differentiate from the paraxial mesoderm in a craniocaudal sequence during the third week. By the end of the fifth week, 42 to 44 pairs of somites are present. The coccygeal somites regress with the tail during the eighth week.

21. **C** Myoblasts from the cervical myotomes form the scalene muscles, as well as the prevertebral, geniohyoid, and infrahyoid muscles.

22. **A** Myoblasts from the pharyngeal arches migrate to form the muscles of mastication (temporalis, masseter, and medial and lateral pterygoids). The muscles of facial expressions, as well as of the pharynx and larynx, are also formed from the myoblasts of the pharyngeal arches. Muscles derived from any one of the pharyngeal arches retain the nerve supply of that particular arch; that is, the trigeminal nerve (CN V) innervates the muscles of mastication, as well as other muscles (mylohyoid, anterior belly of digastric, tensor tympani, tensor veli palatini) that are derived from the first pharyngeal (mandibular) arch. The facial nerve (CN VII), which is the second pharyngeal arch nerve, innervates the muscles of facial expression.

23. **D** The limb muscles are derived from the somites. Grafting and gene targeting studies in birds and mammals indicate that the precursor myogenic cells in limb buds originate from the somites. These cells are first located in the ventral part of the dermomyotome and are epithelial in nature. Following mesenchymal epithelial transformation, the cells then migrate into the anlage or primordium of the limb. The molecular mechanisms involved remain largely unknown.

■ NOTES

Limbs 16

Objectives
Be able to:

- Describe the development of the limbs.
- Define and illustrate the apical ectodermal ridge.
- Describe the development of the bones and muscles of the limbs.
- Describe the effects of teratogens on limb development.
- Construct and label diagrams showing rotation of the limbs.
- Discuss and illustrate the development of the dermatomal patterns of the limbs.

■ FIVE-CHOICE COMPLETION QUESTIONS

Directions: Each of the following statements or questions is followed by five suggested responses or completions. **Select the one best answer** in each case.

1. Teratogens acting after the _____ week will not cause severe limb defects.
   - A. fourth
   - B. fifth
   - C. sixth
   - D. seventh
   - E. eighth

2. Each of the following statements about the apical ectodermal ridge is correct *except*:
   - A. It first appears in the upper limb bud.
   - B. It exerts an inductive influence on the limb mesenchyme.
   - C. It appears at the proximal end of the limb bud.
   - D. It promotes growth and development of the limb.
   - E. Injury to it results in severe limb defects.

3. Each of the following bones develops by endochondral ossification, *except* the
   - A. humerus
   - B. radius
   - C. clavicle
   - D. ulna
   - E. tibia

4. Which of the following bones develops by intramembranous ossification?
   - A. Humerus
   - B. Ulna
   - C. Radius
   - D. Phalanges
   - E. None of the above

Five-Choice Completion Questions *Continued*

5. Congenital clubfoot was diagnosed in a child. In this condition, which of the following statements is correct?
   A. The bones have fused
   B. Involves the talus
   C. The foot is everted
   D. More common in females
   E. The calcaneus is absent

6. With respect to congenital dislocation of the hip, all of the following are correct *except:*
   A. It is more common in females than in males.
   B. Dislocation of the hip occurs in utero.
   C. The acetabulum is underdeveloped.
   D. It occurs in about 1 in 1500 births.
   E. Hereditary factors are involved.

7. For a teratogen to cause absence of the hand, it would have to act before the end of the _____ week.
   A. fifth
   B. sixth
   C. seventh
   D. eighth
   E. ninth

8. With respect to polydactyly, all of the following are correct *except:*
   A. Supernumerary digits are common.
   B. It is inherited as a dominant trait.
   C. In the hand, the extra digit is most commonly central.
   D. In the foot, the extra digit is usually located on the lateral side.
   E. The extra digit may lack proper muscular development.

9. Ossification of the long bones of the limbs begins in the _____ week.
   A. sixth
   B. seventh
   C. eighth
   D. ninth
   E. tenth

10. A full-term infant was born with varying degrees of "webbing" between the fingers. All of the following with respect to this condition are correct *except:*
    A. It occurs in about 1 in 3000 newborns.
    B. It is the most common limb anomaly.
    C. It is inherited as a dominant trait.
    D. It is inherited as a recessive trait.
    E. It results from failure of the digital rays to degenerate.

■ ANSWERS AND EXPLANATIONS

1. **C** By the end of the sixth week, the digital rays of the fingers and toes are differentiated; hence, after this period, teratogenic substances (e.g., drugs) are unable to produce major congenital anomalies (e.g., meromelia—partial absence of a limb).

2. **C** The apical ectodermal ridge appears at the distal end of the limb bud. There is strong evidence of inductor activity by the ridge on the mesenchyme in the limb.

3. **C** The clavicle (part of the pectoral or shoulder girdle) begins to develop by intramenbranous ossification; however, it later develops growth cartilages at each end that give rise to most of the bone by endochondrial ossification.

4. **E** All of these limb bones form by endochondral ossification. Mesenchymal models of the bones form, and chondrification results in cartilage models. Later, bone forms.

5. **B** Any deformity of the foot that involves the talus or ankle bone is known as a clubfoot. In talipes equinovarus, which is the most common type of clubfoot and far more common in males than in females, the sole is turned medially and the foot is inverted. It is believed that both hereditary factors and in utero compression of the fetal lower limbs are responsible for this deformity.

6. **B** Dislocation of the hip almost always occurs after birth. Acetabular insufficiency, laxity of the joint, and hereditary factors usually are involved in the development of this deformity. A higher risk of occurrence exists among siblings because joint laxity often is dominantly inherited.

7. **A** The potent teratogen (thalidomide) known to cause limb defects did not induce absence of the hand when it was ingested later than the 33rd day after the last normal menstrual period. During the sixth to eighth week, only minor limb defects (e.g., hypoplasia of the thumb) can be produced by a teratogenic agent.

8. **C** In polydactyly, one or more extra digits may be present. The condition is a dominant trait and usually runs in families. If the hand is affected, the extra digit is most commonly lateral or medial rather than central. In the foot, the extra digit is usually located on the lateral side. The extra digit is often incompletely formed and lacks proper muscular development. It is now common practice to surgically remove the extra digit after birth.

9. **B** Ossification of the long bones of the limbs begins in the seventh week from primary ossification centers in the middle of the cartilaginous models of the long bones. Cartilage formation in the limbs begins during the fifth week from the mesenchymal models of the bones, and by the end of the sixth week the entire limb skeleton is cartilaginous.

10. **E** Cutaneous syndactyly (simple webbing of the digits) is the most common limb anomaly. This defect is found in about 1 in 3000 newborns. In more serious cases, there is fusion of the digits. Syndactyly is inherited as a simple dominant or simple recessive trait. Cutaneous syndactyly results when the web between two or more digits fails to degenerate. Fusion of the bones (osseous syndactyly) occurs when the notches between the digital rays fail to develop during the seventh week. The digital rays are formed by mesenchymal condensations and represent the primordia of the future digits.

■ FIVE-CHOICE ASSOCIATION QUESTIONS

Directions: Each group of questions below consists of a numbered list of descriptive words or phrases accompanied by a diagram with certain parts indicated by letters or by a list of lettered headings. For each numbered word or phrase, **select the lettered part or heading** that matches it correctly, and then insert the letter in the space to the right of the appropriate number. Sometimes more than one numbered word or phrase may be correctly matched to the same lettered part or heading.

A. Upper limb bud
B. Apical ectodermal ridge
C. Somites
D. Meromelia
E. Lower limb bud

A. Dermatome
B. Phocomelia
C. Digital rays
D. End of fourth week
E. Amelia

1. _____ Partial absence of a limb
2. _____ Limb muscles
3. _____ Rotates medially
4. _____ Rotates laterally
5. _____ Exerts an inductive influence
6. _____ Thalidomide ingestion
7. _____ Condensations of mesenchyme
8. _____ Lower limb bud
9. _____ Area of skin supplied by a spinal nerve
10. _____ Absence of the limbs
11. _____ Type of meromelia

■ ANSWERS AND EXPLANATIONS

1. **D** Meromelia (from Greek *meros,* part, and *melos,* extremity) is the term now used to classify all limb anomalies that involve partial absence of a limb or limbs—for example, *hemimelia* (absence of all or part of the distal half of a limb) and *phocomelia* (absence of the proximal part of a limb or limbs).

2. **C** The limb muscles develop from mesenchyme that is derived from mesenchyme in the myotome regions of the somites. Following mesenchymal epithelial transformation, the muscle forming cells—*myoblasts*—migrate into the primordia of the limbs.

3. **E** The developing lower limbs rotate medially through almost 90 degrees. As a result, the knees face anterolaterally.

4. **A** The developing upper limbs rotate laterally through 90 degrees on their longitudinal axes; as a result, the elbows face dorsally or posteriorly.

5. **B** The apical ectodermal ridge is a thickened, epithelial plaque at the distal end of each limb bud. This ridge is an inducer of limb growth. There is no further elaboration of distal structures (hands and fingers) if the ridge is removed experimentally.

6. **D** Meromelia or partial absence of the limbs commonly was observed in the infants of mothers who ingested thalidomide during the most critical period of limb development (fourth and fifth weeks).

7. **C** The digital rays are condensations of mesenchyme in the hand and foot plates that indicate where the digits will develop.

Answers, Notes, and Explanations *Continued*

8. **D** The lower limb buds appear at the end of the fourth week as ventrolateral outgrowths of the body wall.

9. **A** A dermatome is the area of skin supplied by a single spinal nerve and its spinal ganglion (dorsal root ganglion).

10. **E** Amelia refers to absence of the limbs. This condition resulted when thalidomide was ingested by pregnant women early in the fourth week after fertilization.

11. **B** Phocomelia is a type of meromelia (partial absence of the limbs). In this type of meromelia, the limbs have a flipper-like appearance.

■ NOTES

Nervous System 17

Objectives

Be able to:

- Construct and label diagrams showing early development of the nervous system.
- Define neural plate, neural groove, neural folds, neural crest, neuropores, and primary and secondary brain vesicles.
- Make a simple diagram showing the development of neurons and neuroglial cells.
- Construct and label diagrams showing the brain flexures and indicating the adult derivatives of the walls and cavities of the forebrain, midbrain, and hindbrain.
- Prepare sketches showing the development of the hypophysis cerebri (pituitary gland).
- Discuss the following congenital anomalies of the central nervous system, using sketches as required: meroanencephaly, microcephaly, encephalocele, cranial meningocele, Arnold-Chiari anomaly, spina bifida with meningocele, and spina bifida with meningomyelocele.

■ FIVE-CHOICE COMPLETION QUESTIONS

Directions: Each of the following statements or questions is followed by five suggested responses or completions. **Select the one best answer** in each case.

1. The rostral and caudal neuropores usually close during the _____ week.
   - A. third
   - B. fourth
   - C. fifth
   - D. sixth
   - E. seventh

2. The pons and cerebellum are derived from the walls of the
   - A. hindbrain
   - B. mesencephalon
   - C. myelencephalon
   - D. midbrain
   - E. metencephalon

3. The myelin sheaths surrounding axons in the central nervous system are formed by
   - A. neuroglial cells
   - B. astrocytes
   - C. oligodendrocytes
   - D. microglial cells
   - E. Schwann cells

Five-Choice Completion Questions *Continued*

4. Each of the following cells in the central nervous system is derived from neuroepithelial cells *except*:
   A. ependymal cells
   B. microglial cells
   C. astroglia
   D. motor neurons
   E. choroid epithelial cells

5. Each of the following cells is derived from the neural crest *except*:
   A. melanocytes
   B. Schwann cells
   C. ependymal cells
   D. chromaffin cells
   E. spinal ganglion cells

6. The brain flexure that develops between the metencephalon and the myelencephalon is the _____ flexure.
   A. pontine
   B. cervical
   C. hindbrain
   D. midbrain
   E. cerebellar

7. The neurolemma and myelin sheath of a peripheral nerve fiber are formed by
   A. mesenchymal cells
   B. microglia
   C. neural cells
   D. Schwann cells
   E. neuroepithelial cells

8. The longitudinal groove in the internal surface of the developing spinal cord is called the
   A. neural groove
   B. cuneate groove
   C. sulcus limitans
   D. sulcus longitudinalis
   E. longitudinal groove

9. Each of the following is a derivative of the alar plates *except*:
   A. gracile nucleus
   B. pontine nucleus
   C. dorsal gray horn
   D. cuneate nucleus
   E. ventral gray horn

10. Which of the following structures is *not* a derivative of the diencephalon?
    A. Thalamus
    B. Adenohypophysis
    C. Hypothalamus
    D. Neurohypophysis
    E. Epithalamus

11. The formation of myelin sheaths is largely completed by the end of the _____ period.
    A. embryonic
    B. fetal
    C. perinatal
    D. neonatal
    E. infantile

12. The pineal body develops as a diverticulum of the roof of the
    A. telencephalon
    B. diencephalon
    C. forebrain
    D. mesencephalon
    E. midbrain

Five-Choice Completion Questions *Continued*

13. At birth, the caudal end of the spinal cord lies at the level of the _____ vertebra.
   A. third sacral
   B. first sacral
   C. third lumbar
   D. first lumbar
   E. twelfth thoracic

14. Which of the following may follow infection with cytomegalovirus or *Toxoplasma gondii* during the fetal period?
   A. Mental retardation
   B. Hydrocephaly
   C. Microcephaly
   D. Microphthalmia
   E. All the above

15. Which of the following congenital anomalies of the central nervous system is shown?

   A. Spina bifida with meningocele
   B. Spina bifida cystica
   C. Spina bifida occulta
   D. Spina bifida with myeloschisis
   E. Spina bifida with meningomyelocele

16. At autopsy, a female infant was described as having a major congenital anomaly resulting from failure of the rostral neuropore to close. This condition is known as
   A. spina bifida
   B. meningocele
   C. myeloschisis
   D. meroanencephaly
   E. hydrocephalus

17. A neonate was diagnosed as having a noncommunicating hydrocephalus. Which of the following might have led to this condition?
   A. Obstruction in the circulation of cerebrospinal fluid (CSF)
   B. Excess production of CSF
   C. Increased size of the head
   D. Disturbances in the resorption of CSF
   E. Failure of the neural tube to close

18. Agenesis of the corpus callosum was diagnosed in an infant. Which of the following statements about this condition is (are) correct?
   A. The cause of agenesis of the corpus callosum is not known.
   B. The corpus callosum may be partially absent.
   C. The condition may be asymptomatic.
   D. The corpus callosum may be completely absent.
   E. All of the above.

■ ANSWERS AND EXPLANATIONS

1. **B** The cranial opening in the neural tube, called the rostral neuropore, closes at about 26 days, and the caudal neuropore closes about 2 days later. Failure of the neural folds to fuse and form the forebrain vesicle, or failure of the rostral neuropore to close, results in meroanencephaly (anencephaly). The brain is represented by a mass of largely degenerated nervous tissue. Failure of the neural folds to fuse into the neural tube in the region that gives rise to the spinal cord, or failure of the caudal neuropore to close, results in spina bifida cystica (e.g., spina bifida with meningocele).

2. **E** The walls of the metencephalon give rise to the pons and cerebellum; its cavity forms the superior part of the fourth ventricle. If you chose answer **A**, you were partly correct because the metencephalon is the rostral part of the hindbrain. Answer **E** is more specific; thus, it is the better of the two answers.

3. **C** Oligodendrocytes are responsible for the formation of myelin sheaths in the central nervous system in the same way that Schwann cells form the myelin sheaths of peripheral nerve fibers. The plasma membrane of an oligodendrocyte becomes wrapped around a fiber. The number of layers that are wrapped around the fiber determines the thickness of the myelin sheath. If you selected choice **A**, you were partly right because oligodendrocytes are a type of neuroglial cell. Choice **C** is more specific; thus, it is the better of the two answers.

4. **B** The microglial cells (microglia), scattered through the gray and white matter of the central nervous system, are derived from mesoderm. They invade the central nervous system late in fetal development. To indicate their mesodermal origin, sometimes this type of neuroglial cell is called a mesoglial cell.

5. **C** Ependymal cells, often classified as a type of neuroglial cell, are derived from the neuroepithelium of the neural tube. After the production of neuroblasts (developing neurons) has ceased, the neuroepithelial cells lining the ventricles and the central canal of the spinal cord form the ependymal epithelium or ependyma. Throughout most of the ventricular surface, the ependymal cells have cilia that project into the ventricles. The ependyma that covers the capillaries of the choroid plexuses is of the cuboidal type and called the choroid plexus epithelium.

6. **A** The pontine flexure causes the lateral walls of the medulla to fall outward or laterally like the pages of an opening book. This causes the roof plate to become stretched and the cavity of the hindbrain (future fourth ventricle) to become somewhat rhomboidal or diamond-shaped.

7. **D** The neurolemma and myelin sheath are both components of Schwann cells derived from the neural crest. These cells migrate peripherally and wrap themselves around the fibers of peripheral nerves. One Schwann cell may envelop up to 15 fibers that remain as unmyelinated fibers. Schwann cells ensheathing a single axon develop myelin between the axon and the neurolemma by rotation of the Schwann cell around the axon.

8. **C** The sulcus limitans results from differential thickening of the lateral walls of the developing spinal cord. This sulcus or groove demarcates the dorsal or alar plate (lamina) from the ventral or basal plate (lamina). This regional separation is of fundamental importance because the alar and basal plates are later associated with afferent and efferent functions, respectively.

9. **E** The neurons that form the gray matter in the ventral (anterior) horns of the spinal cord are derived from neuroblasts in the basal plates. The lateral gray columns of the spinal cord are also derived from the basal plates. The alar laminae

Answers and Explanations *Continued*

form the gray columns in the dorsal horns.

10. **B** The adenohypophysis or glandular portion of the hypophysis or pituitary gland is not derived from the diencephalon. It originates from the Rathke pouch, a diverticulum from the roof of the primordial mouth or stomodeum. The neurohypophysis is derived from the infundibulum, a downgrowth from the floor of the diencephalon.

11. **E** Myelination begins during midfetal life (16 to 20 weeks) and is largely completed by the end of the infantile period (12 to 14 months). There are exceptions to these general statements; for example, the descending motor tracts (pyramidal and rubrospinal) do not begin to acquire their myelin sheaths until full term, and the process is not complete until the end of the second year of postnatal life. There is good evidence to indicate that tracts become completely myelinated at about the time they become fully functional.

12. **B** The pineal body (gland), also called the epiphysis, develops as a midline diverticulum of the caudal part of the roof of the diencephalon. It eventually becomes a solid organ located on the roof of the mesencephalon (midbrain). When stimulated, sympathetic fibers in the pineal body release norepinephrine.

13. **C** The caudal or inferior end of the spinal cord usually lies at the level of the third lumbar vertebra in the neonate. This is an average level; it could end as high as the second lumbar vertebra or as low as the fourth lumbar vertebra. In the embryo, the spinal cord extends the entire length of the vertebral canal. Because the vertebral column grows more rapidly than the spinal cord, the cord gradually comes to lie at relatively higher levels. Because a portion of the subarachnoid space extends below the spinal cord (i.e.,

below L3 in the neonate), CSF may be removed without damaging the cord. In the adult, the spinal cord usually ends at the inferior border of the first lumbar vertebra.

14. **E** Maternal infections (cytomegalovirus and *Toxoplasma gondii*) during the fetal period may cause all the congenital abnormalities listed. Rubella infections during the second trimester often produce effects similar to those caused by cytomegalovirus and the parasite *T. gondii,* except that the rubella virus usually causes more severe abnormalities, especially of the eyes and ears.

15. **E** If you chose **B,** you selected the second best answer; it is not as specific as choice **E** because **A** and **D** are also types of spina bifida cystica; that is, they exhibit a saccular protrusion of the spinal cord and/or the meninges.

16. **D** Failure of the rostral or cranial neuropore to close results in meroanencephaly or anencephaly, a clinical condition that is incompatible with postnatal life. It occurs more frequently in female infants.

17. **A** Hydrocephalus is an accumulation of CSF in the ventricular system. There are two types: communicating and noncommunicating. Obstruction in the circulation of CSF leads to a noncommunicating hydrocephalus, and a communicating hydrocephalus results from either excess production or poor resorption of CSF. Increase in the size of the ventricles causes compression and atrophy of the brain, with the head becoming progressively larger. Surgical management of hydrocephalus consists of shunting the CSF from the enlarged lateral ventricles into the pleural or peritoneal cavity.

18. **E** The corpus callosum is the largest cerebral commissure connecting the cerebral hemispheres. It may be partially or

Answers and Explanations *Continued*

completely absent. The cause of this condition is not known, and there is no evidence that it is inherited. Patients with agenesis of the corpus callosum often present without any symptoms and usually have average IQs. Seizures and mental deficiency are not uncommon in cases of agenesis of the corpus callosum.

■ FIVE-CHOICE ASSOCIATION QUESTIONS

Directions: Each group of questions below consists of a numbered list of descriptive words or phrases accompanied by a diagram with certain parts indicated by letters or by a list of lettered headings. For each numbered word or phrase, **select the lettered part or heading** that matches it correctly and then insert the letter in the space to the right of the appropriate number. Sometimes more than one numbered word or phrase may be correctly matched to the same lettered part or heading.

1. _____ Lentiform nucleus
2. _____ Invagination of pia mater
3. _____ Third ventricle
4. _____ Produces CSF
5. _____ Hypothalamus
6. _____ Internal capsule

A. Neural crest cells
B. Alar plates
C. Basal plates
D. Neuroepithelium
E. Spinal ganglion cells

7. _____ Gracile nuclei
8. _____ Form ventral gray columns
9. _____ Sympathetic ganglion cells
10. _____ Neuroglia
11. _____ Efferent function
12. _____ Unipolar afferent neurons

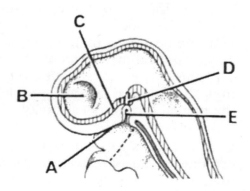

13. _____ Primordium of adenohypophysis
14. _____ Gives rise to the pars nervosa
15. _____ Roof of the primordial mouth cavity
16. _____ Infundibulum
17. _____ Primordium of the cerebral hemisphere
18. _____ Floor of the diencephalon

Five-Choice Association Questions *Continued*

A. Telencephalon
B. Diencephalon
C. Mesencephalon
D. Metencephalon
E. Myelencephalon

19. _____ Pons
20. _____ Olivary nuclei
21. _____ Corpus striatum
22. _____ Thalamus
23. _____ Red nuclei
24. _____ Cerebellum

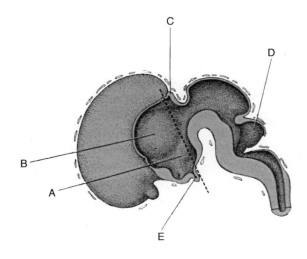

25. _____ Neurohypophysial bud
26. _____ Gives rise to the neurohypophysis
27. _____ Forms the thalamus
28. _____ Includes the mamillary bodies
29. _____ Forms the pineal body
30. _____ Derives from the metencephalon

■ ANSWERS AND EXPLANATIONS

1. **C** As the cerebral cortex differentiates, nerve fibers passing to and from it pass through the swelling called the corpus striatum in the floor of each hemisphere. Soon these fibers divide the corpus striatum into two groups of nerve cells, the caudate and lentiform nuclei.

2. **A** The choroid plexus of the lateral ventricle is formed by an invagination of vascular pia mater, called the tela choroidea, on the medial side of each cerebral hemisphere. The vascular connective tissue acquires a covering layer of epithelium from the ependymal lining of the ventricle.

3. **D** The third ventricle is formed mainly from the cavity of the diencephalon. The extreme anterior part of the third ventricle is derived from the cavity of the telencephalon.

4. **A** The choroid plexuses of the lateral, third, and fourth ventricles produce most of the CSF. The plexuses in the lateral ventricles are the largest and most important producers of CSF. Some CSF is formed by the pia mater on the external surface of the brain.

5. **E** The hypothalamus arises by proliferation of neuroblasts in the ventral wall of the diencephalon. The various nuclei that develop in it are concerned with endocrine activities and homeostasis.

6. **B** As the cerebral cortex differentiates, fibers passing to and from it pass through the corpus striatum; this fiber pathway is called the internal capsule. Projection fibers concentrated in the internal capsule fan out to form the corona radiata in the medullary center. Because of its adaptation to the contours of the masses of gray matter in the brain, the internal cap-

Answers and Explanations *Continued*

sule develops an anterior limb, a genu, and a posterior limb, as seen on horizontal section.

7. **B** The gracile and cuneate nuclei develop from neuroblasts that migrate from the alar plates into the marginal zone of the myelencephalon. These nuclei are associated with correspondingly named tracts that enter the medulla from the spinal cord.

8. **C** The basal plates of the neural tube give rise to the ventral and lateral gray columns of nerve cells in the spinal cord. Axons of the ventral horn cells grow out of the spinal cord and form the ventral roots of spinal nerves.

9. **A** Sympathetic ganglion cells are derived from neuroblasts that differentiate from neural crest cells. Some sympathetic neuroblasts migrate to the suprarenal (adrenal) glands where they differentiate into chromaffin cells of the suprarenal medulla.

10. **D** Some neuroepithelial cells of the neural tube differentiate into glioblasts (also called spongioblasts). These cells give rise to oligodendroblasts and astroblasts, which eventually become oligodendrocytes and astrocytes. Oligodendrocytes are concerned with the formation of myelin sheaths within the central nervous system, and astrocytes provide nutrition and general support to the developing neurons. The formation of glial cells continues into adult life.

11. **C** Neuroepithelial cells in the basal plates of the developing neural tube give rise to neurons (e.g., the motor neurons in the ventral horns of the spinal cord) that are concerned with efferent activities.

12. **E** The unipolar spinal (dorsal root) ganglion cells arise by differentiation of neural crest cells. First bipolar neuroblasts form and then their processes unite to form unipolar neurons. The central process of this T-shaped axon grows into the spinal cord to form part of a dorsal root; the peripheral process forms part of the dorsal root, which joins the ventral root to form a mixed spinal nerve.

13. **E** The primordium of the adenohypophysis is the Rathke pouch, a diverticulum from the ectodermal roof of the primordial mouth cavity or stomodeum. This diverticulum soon contacts the infundibulum, the primordium of the neurohypophysis.

14. **D** The infundibulum gives rise to the neurohypophysis. The infundibulum appears as a ventral bud or diverticulum of the floor of the diencephalon. Later, nerve fibers from the hypothalamus grow into the developing pars nervosa of the pituitary gland.

15. **A** The epithelial roof of the primordial mouth cavity or stomodeum is derived from ectoderm. As the head folds and the pharyngeal arches form during the fourth week, the surface ectoderm becomes depressed to form the primordial mouth cavity in the center of the facial primordia. The Rathke pouch develops as a dorsal diverticulum of the oral ectoderm.

16. **D** The infundibulum gives rise to the neurohypophysis or pars nervosa of the hypophysis cerebri or pituitary gland. As the posterior pituitary develops, the neuroepithelial cells in the wall of the infundibulum proliferate and differentiate into pituicytes.

17. **B** The lateral diverticulum of the telencephalon, indicated in the drawing, gives rise to the right cerebral hemisphere. As it expands, it covers the diencephalon, midbrain, and hindbrain. It eventually meets the other hemisphere in the midline, flattening their medial surfaces.

Answers and Explanations *Continued*

18. **C** The floor of the diencephalon gives rise to the infundibulum (the primordium of the neurohypophysis) and the mamillary bodies. The infundibulum gives rise to the median eminence, the infundibular stem, and the pars nervosa. The infundibulum initially has a thin wall, but its distal end soon becomes thickened as the neuroepithelial cells proliferate. These cells later differentiate into pituicytes.

19. **D** The pons is derived from the metencephalon. Nerve fibers that connect the cerebral and cerebellar cortices with the spinal cord pass through the marginal layer of the ventral region of the metencephalon. These fibers form a robust band of nerve fibers crossing to the other side. This accounts for the name *pons,* which is a Latin word meaning a bridge. The walls of the metencephalon form the pons and cerebellum, and its cavity forms the superior part of the fourth ventricle.

20. **E** The olivary nuclei in the rostral part of the myelencephalon (open part of the medulla) are derived from neuroblasts that migrate from the alar plates.

21. **A** The corpus striatum appears as a prominent swelling in the floor of each cerebral hemisphere. The hemispheres develop from lateral diverticula of the telencephalon. Because of the presence of the corpus striatum in the floor of the hemisphere, the floor expands more slowly than the thin cortical walls. Consequently, the cerebral hemispheres assume a C shape.

22. **B** The thalamus develops from a swelling on each side of the lateral wall of the diencephalon. As the thalamic swellings enlarge, they bulge into the cavity of the diencephalon (developing third ventricle), reducing it to a narrow cavity. The thalamic swellings often meet and fuse in the midline, forming the interthalamic connexus (massa intermedia), which bridges the cavity of the third ventricle.

23. **C** The red nuclei of the midbrain are derived from neuroblasts that arise from the basal plates of the mesencephalon. The basal plates also give rise to the nuclei of the third and fourth cranial nerves and to neurons of the reticular nuclei.

24. **D** The cerebellum develops from symmetrical thickenings of the rostrodorsal parts of the alar plates of the metencephalon. The cerebellar swellings bulge into the cavity of the metencephalon (future fourth ventricle). These primordia eventually fuse and overgrow the rostral half of the fourth ventricle and overlap the pons and medulla.

25. **B** The neurohypophysial bud develops as a ventral diverticulum of the floor of the diencephalon. This bud enlarges to form the infundibulum, primordium of the median eminence, infundibular stem, and pars nervosa of the pituitary gland.

26. **E** The pituitary gland develops from two sources: an upgrowth of the ectodermal roof of the stomodeum and a downgrowth from the neuroectoderm of the diencephalon, known as the infundibulum or neurohypophysial bud. The neurohypophysis, which consists of the median eminence, infundibular stem, and pars nervosa of the pituitary gland, is derived from the infundibulum.

27. **B** The thalamus develops rapidly in the lateral walls of the third ventricle, reducing it to a narrow cleft. In 70% of brains, the thalami meet and fuse in the midline, forming a bridge of gray matter (the interthalamic adhesion or massa intermedia) across the third ventricle.

28. **A** A pair of nuclei, the mamillary bodies, are located on the ventral surface of the hypothalamus. The hypothalamus arises by proliferation of neuroblasts in the lateral walls of the third ventricle. It

Answers and Explanations *Continued*

is separated from the thalamus by a shallow groove, the hypothalamic sulcus.

29. **C** The pineal body (gland) develops as a median diverticulum from the caudal part of the roof the diencephalon. It is converted into a solid cone-shaped gland by cellular proliferation.

30. **D** The cerebellum is derived from the walls of the metencephalon. The pons also arises from the metencephalon. The cerebellum arises bilaterally from the dorsal parts of the alar plates. The cerebellar primordia enlarge, projecting into the fourth ventricle and eventually fusing in the median plane to form the vermis.

■ NOTES

Objectives

Be able to:

- Construct and label diagrams showing early development of the eyes.
- Define optic sulci, optic vesicles, optic stalks, optic fissures, optic cups, lens placodes, lens pits, and lens vesicles.
- Describe the development of the retina, ciliary body, and iris, using labeled sketches.
- Write brief notes on the formation of the lens, choroid, sclera, cornea, and optic nerve.
- Construct and label diagrams showing the development of the internal ear, middle ear, and external ear.
- Define otic placode, otic pit, otic vesicle, endolymphatic duct and sac, spiral organ (of Corti), and semicircular ducts.
- Discuss the embryological basis of the following congenital anomalies: coloboma, glaucoma, cataract, and deafness.

■ FIVE-CHOICE COMPLETION QUESTIONS

Directions: Each of the following statements or questions is followed by five suggested responses or completions. **Select the one best answer** in each case.

1. Which of the following structures is *not* derived from neuroectoderm?
   A. Epithelium of the iris
   B. Optic nerve
   C. Corneal epithelium
   D. Muscles of the iris
   E. Retina

2. Which of the following structures is *not* derived from mesoderm?
   A. Choroid
   B. Bony labyrinth
   C. Extrinsic eye muscles
   D. Membranous labyrinth
   E. Sclera

3. Structures derived from the surface ectoderm include the
   A. lens
   B. otic vesicle
   C. external acoustic meatus
   D. corneal epithelium
   E. all the above

4. The epithelium of the iris develops from the
   A. inner layer of the rim of the optic cup
   B. outer layer of the rim of the optic cup
   C. both layers of the rim of the optic cup
   D. mesenchyme near the rim of the optic cup
   E. mesenchyme between the lens and the cornea

Five-Choice Completion Questions *Continued*

5. The inner, nonpigmented portion of the ciliary epithelium is continuous with the
   A. neural layer of the retina
   B. sphincter of the pupil
   C. pigmented epithelium of the retina
   D. anterior surface of the iris
   E. corneal epithelium

6. The choroid is derived from the
   A. mesoderm surrounding the eye primordium
   B. loose mesenchyme near the optic cup
   C. mesenchyme from the occipital myotomes
   D. mesenchyme between the sclera and pigmented layer of the retina
   E. mesenchyme from the first pair of pharyngeal arches

7. Cellular components of the retina derived from the inner layer of the optic cup include
   A. rod cells
   B. ganglion cells
   C. neuroglial cells
   D. bipolar cells
   E. all the above

8. During examination of the eyes of a neonate, you noted that one pupil was pear-shaped owing to a defect in the iris. What is the most likely cause of this typical coloboma of the iris?
   A. Genetic factors
   B. Rubella virus
   C. Toxoplasmosis
   D. Radiation
   E. Cytomegalovirus

9. You examine a neonate and diagnose congenital heart disease. You also observe bilateral cataracts. During discussions with the infant's mother, you learn that she had a fever, sore throat, and rash on her face, body, and limbs shortly after her first missed menstrual period. She also recalled taking some tranquilizers and sedatives during early pregnancy to settle her nerves and help her sleep. What do you think would be the most likely cause of the congenital anomalies you have detected in her baby?
   A. Measles (rubeola)
   B. Congenital galactosemia
   C. Teratogenic drugs
   D. Influenza
   E. None of the above

10. The otic vesicle or otocyst gives rise to the
    A. saccule
    B. utricle
    C. cochlear duct
    D. endolymphatic sac
    E. all the above

Five-Choice Completion Questions *Continued*

11. An inferior notch or coloboma of the iris was detected in an infant. This condition probably is caused by which of the following?
    A. Localized disturbance in the development of the lower eyelid
    B. Defective closure of the optic fissure
    C. Congenital glaucoma
    D. Failure of the mesenchyme surrounding the optic cup to differentiate
    E. Degeneration of the pupillary membrane

12. Physical examination of a neonate revealed that the external acoustic meatus is atretic. This condition is the result of which of the following?
    A. Otic pit did not form
    B. Development of the first pharyngeal pouch is affected
    C. Failure of the meatal plug to canalize
    D. Auricular hillocks did not develop
    E. Tubotympanic recess has degenerated

■ ANSWERS AND EXPLANATIONS

1. **C** The cornea has a dual origin: the stratified squamous, nonkeratinizing epithelium is derived from the surface ectoderm; the substantia propria and other parts of the cornea are derived from mesoderm. Muscles usually are derived from mesoderm. The dilator and sphincter pupillae muscles of the iris are exceptions; they are derived from the neuroectoderm of the outer layer of the optic cup.

2. **D** The membranous labyrinth is derived from the otic vesicle (otocyst), which develops from an invagination of the surface ectoderm. The otic vesicle soon loses its connection with the surface (future skin).

3. **E** All these structures are derived from the surface ectoderm. The lens develops from the lens vesicle; the otic vesicle gives rise to the membranous labyrinth; the external acoustic meatus develops from the first groove; and the corneal epithelium arises directly from the surface ectoderm. Other parts of the cornea are derived from mesoderm.

4. **C** The double-layered, pigmented epithelium of the iris develops from the inner and outer layers of the rim of the optic cup. Because this epithelium is continuous with the ciliary epithelium and the retina, it often is wrongly assumed to be homologous only to the pigmented layers of these structures derived from the outer layer of the optic cup.

5. **A** The ciliary epithelium is composed of two layers of cells derived from the continuation of the two layers of the retina. The cells of the inner, nonpigmented portion of the ciliary epithelium are continuous with the neural layer of the retina. They become heavily pigmented, however, in the iridial portion of the retina.

6. **D** Three of these answers are correct (**A**, **B**, and **D**) but **D** is the best answer because it is the most specific. The mesenchyme surrounding the optic cup differentiates into an inner vascular layer, the choroid, and an outer fibrous layer, the sclera.

7. **E** All these cells are derived from the inner layer of the optic cup. The rod photo-

Answers and Explanations *Continued*

receptor cells are more numerous than the cone photoreceptors. The bipolar cells are true neurons interposed between the photoreceptor cells and the ganglion cells. The inner layers of the retina, in particular, contain neuroglial cells similar to those in the gray matter of the brain.

8. **A** Most cases of coloboma of the iris are genetically determined with dominant transmission. Some colobomas are associated with maternal infections (including rubella and toxoplasmosis), and it is possible that these and other teratogenic factors may produce colobomas because their development can be induced experimentally in animals. The embryological basis of a typical coloboma of the iris is failure of the optic fissure on the inferior surface of the optic cup to close. Closure of this fissure typically occurs during the sixth week.

9. **E** None of the factors listed probably caused the anomalies exhibited by the infant. The most likely cause of these abnormalities was a maternal rubella (German measles) infection during early pregnancy. The infant exhibited two of the common abnormalities of the *congenital rubella syndrome* (congenital heart defects and cataracts). Congenital galactosemia could produce the cataracts, but this is an uncommon cause. Tranquilizers are not known to cause anomalies, and thalidomide is the only sedative known to be teratogenic. Influenza and rubeola are not known to be causes of congenital anomalies.

10. **E** All these structures are derived from the otic vesicle (otocyst), derived from the surface ectoderm. The cochlear duct contains the spiral organ (of Corti), the receptor of auditory stimuli. The other parts of the membranous labyrinth, derived from the otic vesicle, contain sensory areas of the vestibular system.

11. **B** Coloboma of the iris is caused by a defect in the closure of the optic fissure. This typically occurs during the sixth week. Coloboma of the iris often is associated with other ocular defects. Coloboma of the eyelid is probably caused by a localized disturbance during development of the lid.

12. **C** Atresia of the external acoustic meatus canal is a relatively common condition. It often is unilateral and associated with abnormalities of the auricle. Failure of the meatal plug of the first pharyngeal groove to canalize leads to atresia of the external acoustic meatus. This anomaly usually results from autosomal dominant inheritance.

■ FIVE-CHOICE ASSOCIATION QUESTIONS

Directions: Each group of questions below consists of a numbered list of descriptive words or phrases accompanied by a diagram with certain parts indicated by letters or by a list of lettered headings. For each numbered word or phrase, **select the lettered part or heading** that matches it correctly and then insert the letter in the space to the right of the appropriate number. Sometimes more than one numbered word or phrase may be correctly matched to the same lettered part or heading.

A. Sinus venosus sclerae
B. Optic nerve
C. Corneal epithelium
D. Central artery of retina
E. Pupillary membrane

1. _____ Becomes pigmented layer of the retina
2. _____ Optic fissure
3. _____ Becomes specialized for sensitivity to light
4. _____ Gives rise to the lens
5. _____ Future optic nerve
6. _____ Differentiates into nonpigmented portion of the ciliary epithelium

7. _____ Tunica vasculosa lentis
8. _____ Ganglion cells of the retina
9. _____ Hyaloid artery
10. _____ Surface ectoderm
11. _____ Congenital glaucoma
12. _____ Neuroectoderm

A. Conjunctival epithelium
B. Neuroectoderm
C. First pharyngeal pouch
D. First branchial groove
E. Mesenchyme

13. _____ Gives rise to a semicircular duct
14. _____ Absorption focus
15. _____ Endolymphatic duct
16. _____ Primordium of the cochlea
17. _____ Saccular portion of the otic vesicle
18. _____ Gives rise to the spiral organ

19. _____ External acoustic meatus
20. _____ Sclera and choroid
21. _____ Has same origin as cornea
22. _____ Mastoid cells
23. _____ Bipolar cells of the retina
24. _____ Tympanic cavity

Five-Choice Association Questions *Continued*

level of section

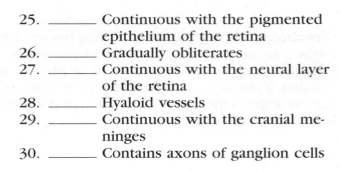

25. _____ Continuous with the pigmented epithelium of the retina
26. _____ Gradually obliterates
27. _____ Continuous with the neural layer of the retina
28. _____ Hyaloid vessels
29. _____ Continuous with the cranial meninges
30. _____ Contains axons of ganglion cells

31. _____ Derived from the Meckel cartilage
32. _____ Gives rise to the utricle
33. _____ External acoustic meatus
34. _____ Meatal plug
35. _____ Derived from the tubotympanic recess
36. _____ Membranous labyrinth

37. _____ Derived from surface ectoderm
38. _____ Ciliary body
39. _____ Develops from mesenchyme
40. _____ Composed of vitreous humor
41. _____ Cornea

■ ANSWERS AND EXPLANATIONS

1. **B** The external layer of the optic cup differentiates into the pigmented layer of the retina. The pigmented epithelium consists of a single layer of cells that reinforces the light-absorbing properties of the choroid membrane to reduce scattering of light within the eye.

2. **E** The optic fissure (choroidal or fetal fissure) develops on the inferior (caudal) surface of the optic cup and along the optic stalk. The hyaloid blood vessels pass into the optic cup along this groove and supply the lens and the developing neural layer of the retina.

3. **C** The inner layer of the optic cup becomes the pars optica retinae or the neural layer of the retina. It differentiates into the visual receptive portion of the adult retina. The inner layer of the optic cup also gives rise to the pars ciliaris retinae and the pars iridis retinae.

4. **D** The lens develops from the lens vesicle, a derivative of the surface ectoderm. The anterior wall of this vesicle becomes the anterior epithelium of the adult lens. Cells of the posterior wall lengthen to form lens fibers, which grow into and gradually obliterate the cavity of the lens vesicle.

5. **A** The optic stalk, connecting the optic cup to the brain, becomes the optic nerve as axons of ganglion cells in the neural layer of the retina pass into the inner wall of the stalk. As a result of the continually increasing number of optic nerve fibers, the inner wall of the stalk increases in thickness and fuses with the outer wall, obliterating the lumen of the optic stalk.

6. **C** Most of the inner layer of the optic cup becomes the neural layer of the retina. The anterior part becomes the nonpigmented portion of the ciliary epithelium (ciliary portion of the retina) and the iridial portion of the retina. Toward the root of the iris, on the anterior surface of the ciliary processes, the cells of the inner layer of the cup gradually accumulate pigment granules.

7. **E** The anterior portion of the tunica vasculosa lentis, a vascular layer around the embryonic lens, is called the pupillary membrane. When the distal portion of the hyaloid artery degenerates, the tunica vasculosa lentis, including the pupillary membrane, also degenerate. Remnants of this membrane often appear as tissue strands in normal eyes of infants, but these strands usually cause little disturbance of vision and tend to disappear in old age.

8. **B** As the neural layer of the retina develops from the inner layer of the optic cup, the axons of ganglion cells in the retina pass into the inner wall of the optic stalk and gradually convert it into the optic nerve.

9. **D** The hyaloid artery passes along the optic fissure to the optic cup, where it supplies blood to the developing neural layer of the retina and to the embryonic lens. The distal portion of this artery usually degenerates, but the proximal portion persists as the central artery of the retina. Persistence of the distal portion of the hyaloid artery is a fairly common abnormality. It may persist in whole or in part, but it usually is not patent. The hyaloid arterial remnant appears as a thin line or thick cord in the vitreous humor (body).

10. **C** The corneal epithelium is derived from the surface ectoderm. The lens functions as an inductor and influences the surface ectoderm to develop into the epithelium of the cornea. The substantia propria of the cornea is derived from mesenchyme.

11. **A** Absence or incomplete development of the sinus venosus sclerae (canal of

Answers and Explanations *Continued*

Schlemm) results in congenital glaucoma or buphthalmos. This abnormality usually is caused by recessive mutant genes, but sometimes it results from a maternal rubella infection during early pregnancy. The embryological basis of blockage or incomplete development of the canal of Schlemm is abnormal persistence of mesenchymal tissue in the angle of the anterior chamber. As a result of inadequate drainage of the aqueous humor through the canal, intraocular tension rises, the eye gradually enlarges, and the cornea becomes hazy. Retinal damage causes visual impairment.

12. **B**   The optic vesicle is an outgrowth of the brain. Hence, the retina and the optic nerve are derived from neuroectoderm of the embryonic brain. The adult structure of the retina and optic nerve shows a marked resemblance to the brain, and the coats of the eyeball and the optic nerve show resemblances to the coverings of the brain. The central artery and vein of the retina pass in the meningeal sheaths and are included in the anterior part of the optic nerve. This relation is of clinical significance because an increase in pressure of cerebrospinal fluid around the optic nerve interferes with venous return from the eye, and edema of the optic disc (papilledema) results. This is an important indicator of an increase in intracranial pressure.

13. **C**   This flat, disclike diverticulum of the dorsal or utricular portion of the otic vesicle is the primordium of one of the three semicircular ducts. They are attached to the utricle and later are enclosed in the semicircular canals of the bony labyrinth. The sensory areas (cristae ampullares), which develop in these ducts, respond to changes in the direction of movement of the head.

14. **E**   The central portions of the walls of the disclike diverticula from the utricular portion of the otocyst fuse and later dis-

appear. Degeneration of tissue proceeds peripherally from the absorption focus, but peripheral portions of the diverticula remain as the semicircular ducts. As the bony labyrinth forms around the ducts, they come to lie in semicircular canals.

15. **D**   The endolymphatic duct appears as a hollow diverticulum from the dorsal utricular portion of the otocyst. Its distal end expands to form the endolymphatic sac.

16. **A**   The cochlear duct develops as a tubular diverticulum from the saccular portion of the otocyst. The cochlear duct grows and makes two and a half turns around the developing modiolus, a bony pillar or core that contains nerves and vessels. The coiled cochlear duct is called the membranous cochlea. It is contained in the bony cochlea, which develops from the surrounding mesenchyme.

17. **B**   The saccular portion of the otic vesicle, called the saccule, is an endolymph-containing dilation of the membranous labyrinth. The saccule contains a specialized area of sensory epithelium, the macula sacculi, and together with the macula utriculi signals the orientation of the head in space.

18. **A**   The spiral organ (of Corti) differentiates from cells in the wall of the cochlear duct. Ganglion cells of the eighth cranial nerve migrate along the coils of the cochlea and form the cochlear (spiral) ganglion. Nerve processes grow from this ganglion to the spiral organ.

19. **D**   The external acoustic meatus is the adult derivative of the dorsal part of the first pharyngeal groove. It grows inward as a funnel-shaped tube until it reaches the endodermal tubotympanic recess, primordium of the tympanic cavity, tympanic antrum, pharyngotympanic (auditory) tube, and mastoid cells.

20. **E**   The sclera and choroid develop from mesenchyme that surrounds the optic

Answers and Explanations *Continued*

cup. The mesenchyme differentiates into an inner vascular layer, the choroid, and an outer fibrous layer, the sclera. Toward the margin of the optic cup, the choroid becomes modified to form the cores of the ciliary processes, which consist chiefly of capillaries supported by delicate connective tissue.

21. **A** The conjunctival epithelium, like the corneal epithelium, is derived from the surface ectoderm. The substantia (lamina) propria of the conjunctiva and cornea consists of connective tissue derived from mesenchyme. The conjunctiva is a thin, transparent mucous membrane that covers the sclera and lines the eyelid. At the lid margin, the epithelium of the conjunctiva becomes continuous with the epidermis of the skin, another derivative of the surface ectoderm.

22. **C** The mastoid cells begin to develop near term as the endodermal lining of the tympanic cavity, a derivative of the first pharyngeal pouch, induces erosion of the bone around the ear. The epithelium lining the mastoid cells formed by this process, called pneumatization, is derived from endoderm. Most mastoid cells develop after birth.

23. **B** The bipolar cells of the neural portion of the retina are derived from neuroectoderm of the brain. These cells are true neurons interposed between photoreceptor cells and ganglion cells.

24. **C** The tympanic cavity develops from the expanded distal end of the tubotympanic recess, a derivative of the first pharyngeal pouch. The tympanic cavity is a tiny epithelium-lined cavity in bone that communicates with the nasopharynx through the pharyngotympanic tube, another derivative of the first pharyngeal pouch.

25. **B** The outer wall of the optic stalk is continuous with the outer wall of the op-

tic cup, which gives rise to the pigmented epithelium of the retina.

26. **A** The lumen of the optic stalk gradually obliterates as the optic nerve forms. As the number of axons of ganglion cells from the retina increases in the inner wall of the optic stalk, the lumen gradually disappears and the optic nerve forms.

27. **D** The internal layer of the optic stalk is continuous with the inner layer of the optic cup, which gives rise to the neural layer of the retina. The internal layer of the optic stalk thickens as axons of ganglion cells pass through it on their way to the brain.

28. **E** The hyaloid vessels supply blood to and return blood from the inner layer of the optic cup (future neural layer of retina) and the embryonic lens. The distal portions of these vessels usually degenerate and the remaining parts become the central artery and vein of the retina. When the optic fissure closes, these vessels are incorporated into the optic nerve.

29. **C** The sheath of the optic nerve is continuous with the meninges of the brain and with the choroid and sclera. When the optic vesicles develop as outgrowths of the brain, they carry the layers of the meninges with them.

30. **D** The internal layer of the optic stalk contains axons of ganglion cells in the neural layer of the retina. About 1 million fibers eventually pass through the optic nerve, the adult derivative of the optic stalk. The optic nerve fibers are myelinated by oligodendrocytes instead of by Schwann cells because the optic nerve is comparable to a tract within the brain. The neuroepithelial cells in the walls of the optic stalk differentiate into oligodendrocytes and other neuroglial cells.

Answers and Explanations *Continued*

31. **C** The malleus, one of the middle ear bones or auditory ossicles, is derived from the first pharyngeal arch cartilage or Meckel cartilage. It develops by endochondral ossification of the dorsal end of the cartilage. The incus and stapes, the other two ossicles, are derived in a similar manner from the first and second branchial arch cartilages, respectively.

32. **D** The dorsal or utricular portion of the otic vesicle (otocyst) gives rise to the utricle. Like the saccule, it is a dilation of the membranous labyrinth that contains a specialized area of sensory epithelium, the macula utriculi. The utricle and saccule are sensors of head movements.

33. **B** The external acoustic meatus is the adult derivative of the dorsal end of the first pharyngeal groove. This canal leads to the tympanic membrane, and its function (along with the auricle) is to collect sound waves, which cause resonant vibration of the tympanic membrane.

34. **A** The ectodermal cells at the bottom of the developing external acoustic meatus proliferate and grow caudally as a solid epithelial plate called the meatal plug. Late in fetal life, the central cells of this plug degenerate, forming the inner portion of the external acoustic meatus. Failure of the meatal plug to canalize results in atresia of the external acoustic meatus and deafness. This condition usually is caused by genetic factors.

35. **E** The pharyngotympanic (auditory) tube is derived from the tubotympanic recess, the derivative of the first pharyngeal pouch. This tube makes possible adjustments of pressure in the middle ear. When the tube opens during swallowing, the pressure in the middle ear becomes equalized with the atmospheric pressure.

36. **D** The membranous labyrinth develops from the otic vesicle, a derivative of the surface ectoderm. It gives rise to the utricle, saccule, endolymphatic duct and sac, semicircular ducts, and cochlea. The internal ear, which has a dual function (hearing and equilibrium), consists of the membranous labyrinth derived from the otic vesicle. It is enclosed in the bony labyrinth derived from the surrounding mesenchyme.

37. **D** The lens develops from the lens vesicle, a derivative of the surface ectoderm. The anterior wall of the hollow lens vesicle, composed of cuboidal epithelium, becomes the anterior lens epithelium. The tall columnar cells of the posterior wall of the vesicle lengthen to form highly transparent primary lens fibers that gradually fill the cavity of the vesicle. In congenital cataract, the lens of the eye is opaque, resulting in blindness.

38. **B** The pigmented region of the epithelium of the ciliary body is derived from the outer region of the optic cup. It is continuous with the retinal pigment epithelium. The nonpigmented portion of the ciliary epithelium represents the interior prolongation of the neural retina in which no neural elements differentiate. The ciliary muscle and connective tissue in the ciliary body develop from mesenchyme or early fibroblasts found at the edge of the optic cup.

39. **E** The mesenchyme surrounding the optic cup differentiates into an inner vascular layer, the choroid, and an outer fibrous tunic, the sclera. The sclera develops from a condensation of the mesenchyme external to the choroid. It is continuous with the substantia propria of the cornea and with the dura mater that surrounds the optic nerve.

40. **A** The vitreous body forms within the cavity of the optic cup, between the lens and retina. It is composed of vitreous humor, an avascular mass of intercellular substance. The primary vitreous forms

from mesenchymal cells and hyaloid blood vessels. The mesenchymal cells are probably of neural crest origin. The primary vitreous becomes surrounded by a gelatinous secondary vitreous that probably arises from the inner layer of the optic cup. The secondary vitreous is formed from primitive hyalocytes, compact collagenous fibrillar material, and hyaluronic acid.

41. **C** The lens induces formation of the cornea, which develops following separation of the lens vesicle from the surface ectoderm. The anterior surface of the cornea, which is covered by a stratified squamous, nonkeratinizing epithelium, forms from the surface ectoderm. The other layers of the cornea are probably derived from neural crest cells.

■ NOTES

Integumentary System 19

Objectives

Be able to:

- Construct and label diagrams showing the development of skin, hair, nails, and sebaceous, sweat, and mammary glands.
- Write explanatory notes on each of the following congenital anomalies: ichthyosis, ectodermal dysplasia, athelia, amastia, polymastia, and polythelia.
- Discuss the development of teeth using labeled sketches to show the various stages of development.
- Define dental lamina, dental papilla, dental sac, epithelial root sheath, odontoblastic layer, odontoblastic processes, ameloblasts, and cementoblasts.
- Describe eruption of the deciduous and permanent teeth.
- Discuss the various causes of disturbances in enamel formation that result in enamel hypoplasia.

■ FIVE-CHOICE COMPLETION QUESTIONS

Directions: Each of the following statements or questions is followed by five suggested responses or completions. **Select the one best answer** in each case.

1. Each of the following structures is derived from the surface ectoderm *except* the
   - A. dental papilla
   - B. fingernails
   - C. epidermis
   - D. sweat glands
   - E. tooth buds

2. Which structure is *not* derived from mesenchyme?
   - A. Dental sac
   - B. Dermal root sheath
   - C. Arrector pili muscle
   - D. Odontoblastic layer
   - E. Epithelial root sheath

3. Which cells are derived from neuroectoderm?
   - A. Ameloblasts
   - B. Odontoblasts
   - C. Cementoblasts
   - D. Melanoblasts
   - E. Myoblasts

4. Most sebaceous glands develop as
   - A. downgrowths of the stratum germinativum
   - B. thickened areas of the epidermis
   - C. buds from the sides of hair follicles
   - D. downgrowths from the surface ectoderm
   - E. ingrowths along the glandular ridges

Five-Choice Completion Questions *Continued*

5. The ameloblasts of the developing tooth produce

    A. predentin   D. periodontium
    B. dentin   E. enamel
    C. cementum

6. The odontoblasts of the developing tooth produce

    A. predentin   D. periodontium
    B. dentin   E. enamel
    C. cementum

7. Which of the following congenital anomalies is common?

    A. Hypertrichosis   D. Polymastia
    B. Anonychia   E. Anodontia
    C. Ectodermal dysplasia

8. Most congenital anomalies of teeth are caused by

    A. tetracyclines   D. irradiation
    B. genetic factors   E. syphilis
    C. rubella virus

9. "Birth marks" of flat, red cutaneous lesions were present on the face of a 3-month-old infant. This condition, diagnosed as angiomas of the skin, is caused by which of the following?

    A. Increased melanocyte activity
    B. Developmental defect of the dermis
    C. Abnormal differentiation of the epidermis
    D. Vascular anomalies
    E. Excessive keratinization

10. Hypertrichosis was observed in the sacral region of a patient. This condition is associated with which of the following?

    A. Spinal dermal sinus   D. Spina bifida cystica
    B. Arnold-Chiari defect   E. Spina bifida occulta
    C. Absence of the sacral vertebrae

11. The teeth of an 8-year-old child were badly discolored, giving them a brownish yellow appearance, and the enamel was hypoplastic. This condition usually is associated with which of the following?

    A. Congenital syphilis   D. Hypothyroidism
    B. Tetracyclines   E. Dental papilla
    C. Periodontal disease

12. Regarding congenital ectodermal dysplasia, all of the following are correct *except* that

    A. it is not inherited.   D. body hair may be sparse or absent.
    B. the skin is usually lax.   E. the teeth may be absent or defective.
    C. sweat glands may be absent.

Five-Choice Completion Questions *Continued*

13. In generalized albinism, which of the following usually shows some pigmentation?
   A. Retina
   B. Iris
   C. Hair
   D. Skin
   E. None of the above

14. Which of the following is *not* a hereditary disorder?
   A. Localized albinism
   B. Dentinogenesis imperfecta
   C. Hemangiomas
   D. Lamellar ichthyosis
   E. Polymastia

15. Which of the following is (are) involved in the growth of the lactiferous ducts after birth?
   A. Estrogens
   B. Progestogens
   C. Prolactin
   D. Growth hormone
   E. All of the above

16. Regarding melanocytes and melanin, all of the following statements are correct *except*
   A. melanocytes are derived from neural crest cells.
   B. melanocytes produce melanin before birth.
   C. exposure to ultraviolet light increases melanin production.
   D. cells containing melanin are present only in dermis.
   E. melanocytes are unable to produce melanin in the absence of the enzyme tyrosinase.

■ ANSWERS AND EXPLANATIONS

1. **A** The dental papilla is a mass of condensed mesenchyme that invaginates the deep surface of the tooth bud. The dental papilla gives rise to the dentin and dental pulp.

2. **E** The epithelial root sheath of the hair follicle and of the developing tooth is derived from the surface ectoderm. The dermal sheath (connective tissue) of the hair follicle, like the dental sac, is derived from mesenchyme.

3. **D** Melanoblasts are derived from the neural crest, a derivative of the neuroectoderm. When the neural folds fuse to form the neural plate, some cells are not incorporated into it. These cells form a neural crest, which gives rise to the cells in the cranial, spinal, and autonomic ganglia; Schwann cells; melanoblasts; and cells of the suprarenal (adrenal) medulla. If you chose **B**, you could be right because there is evidence suggesting that the odontoblasts differentiate from mesenchyme that is of neural crest origin. **D** is the best answer because it is well established that melanoblasts are of neural crest origin.

4. **C** All sebaceous glands develop as buds from the sides of the developing epithelial root sheaths of hair follicles, except those in the glans penis, eyelids, nostrils, anal region, and labia minora. In these sites, sebaceous glands develop as buds from the epidermis.

Answers and Explanations *Continued*

5. **E** The ameloblasts differentiate from the cells in the inner enamel epithelium of the enamel organ. They produce enamel in the form of prisms (rods) and deposit it over the dentin. Each melanoblast produces one enamel rod, the structural unit of enamel. The ameloblasts degenerate after they have formed all the enamel and the tooth erupts. Thus, enamel is incapable of repair if it is injured by decay or injury.

6. **A** The odontoblasts produce predentin and deposit it adjacent to the inner enamel epithelium. Later, the predentin calcifies and becomes dentin. Hence, **A** is a better answer than **B**.

7. **D** An extra breast (mammary gland), called polymastia, is quite common. About 1% of women have an extra breast or nipple. These usually develop just inferior to the normal breast, but they may appear anywhere along the line of the embryonic mammary ridges that run from the axillae to the inguinal regions.

8. **B** Most congenital anomalies of the teeth are hereditary (i.e., they are caused by genetic factors). The importance of genetic factors in tooth development and dental abnormalities is clearly demonstrated by studying the dentition in monozygotic twins. Tetracycline, an antibiotic, crosses the placenta and causes minor tooth defects (enamel hypoplasia) and discoloration of the deciduous teeth. Rubella virus, *Treponema pallidum* (the syphilis organism), and irradiation may also give rise to abnormalities to the teeth. Nutritional deficiency, diseases such as measles, and *high levels* of fluoride may damage the ameloblasts and cause defective enamel formation (enamel hypoplasia). Rickets resulting from a deficiency of vitamin D is, however, the most common cause of enamel hypoplasia. Abnormally shaped teeth are relatively common. Occasionally aberrant groups of ameloblasts give rise to spheri-

cal masses of enamel, called enamel pearls (drops), which often project from the side of the tooth.

9. **D** Angiomas of the skin or hemangiomas are localized vascular anomalies. A true hemangioma is a benign tumor of proliferating endothelium. These lesions include capillary angioma or cavernous hemangioma, the most common neoplasms found in infants and children.

10. **E** Hypertrichosis, or excessive hairiness, in the sacral area often is found in association with spina bifida occulta. It most commonly is seen over congenital melanocytic nevi. Hypertrichosis results from the development of supernumerary hair follicles and from the persistence of hairs that normally disappear during the perinatal period.

11. **B** Tetracyclines affect enamel formation and become incorporated into the developing enamel. These antibiotics should not be used during pregnancy and in children under age 12 because they interfere with metabolic processes that involve the ameloblasts.

12. **A** This is a rare hereditary disorder resulting from disturbances in the development of the epidermis and its appendages. The skin is defective and appears lax; often, other derivatives of the ectoderm, such as nails, hair, and sebaceous glands, may be partially or completely absent. Different clinical manifestations of ectodermal dysplasias have been recognized. Most likely, several modes of inheritance are possible for this condition.

13. **B** In cases of generalized albinism, the iris usually shows some pigmentation; however, the skin, hair, and retina lack pigment. Because of the lack of the enzyme tyrosinase, melanin is not produced by the melanocytes. In localized albinism, there is a lack of melanin in patches of

Answers and Explanations *Continued*

skin, such as on the face, and/or of the hair.

14. **C** Hemangiomas are vascular anomalies, usually located on the face or neck. They are not an inheritable condition. Localized albinism and dentinogenesis imperfecta are autosomal dominant traits; lamellar ichthyosis is an autosomal recessive disorder; and polymastia (extra breast) is an inheritable condition.

15. **E** The main lactiferous ducts are formed at birth. Further growth and development of the lactiferous ducts in females occur particularly at puberty because of increased levels of circulating estrogens. Progestogens, prolactin, growth hormone, and corticoids also play a role. Increase in size of the female mammary glands during pregnancy is largely due to the rapid enlargement of the lactiferous ducts and deposition of fat.

16. **D** Only a few melanin-containing cells are normally present in the dermis. In the white race, the cell bodies of the melanocytes are usually confined to the basal layers of the epidermis. Melanocytes differentiate from melanoblasts, which are derived from neural crest cells. Melanocytes appear in the developing skin between 40 and 50 days of gestation and begin to produce melanin before birth. Exposure to ultraviolet light results in an increased production of melanin.

■ FIVE-CHOICE ASSOCIATION QUESTIONS

Directions: Each group of questions below consists of a numbered list of descriptive words or phrases accompanied by a diagram with certain parts indicated by letters or by a list of lettered headings. For each numbered word or phrase, **select the lettered part or heading** that matches it correctly and then insert the letter in the space to the right of the appropriate number. Sometimes more than one numbered word or phrase may be correctly matched to the same lettered part or heading.

A. Dental pulp
B. Predentin
C. Dental sac
D. Enamel
E. Cementum

1. _____ Periodontal ligament
2. _____ Odontoblasts
3. _____ Inner enamel epithelium
4. _____ Contains vessels and nerves
5. _____ Ameloblasts
6. _____ Inner cells of dental sac

7. _____ Inner enamel epithelium
8. _____ Dental sac
9. _____ Dental lamina
10. _____ Dental papilla
11. _____ Bud of permanent tooth
12. _____ Part of the enamel organ

Five-Choice Association Questions *Continued*

A. Tetracyclines
B. Ameloblastic layer
C. Hair follicles
D. Neural crest cells
E. Epithelial root sheath of the developing
   tooth

13. _____ Melanocytes
14. _____ Induction of odontoblastic layer
15. _____ Lanugo
16. _____ Discoloration of the teeth
17. _____ Sebaceous glands
18. _____ Fused layers of enamel epithelia
19. _____ Derived from the inner enamel
            epithelium
20. _____ Derived from the neural plate

■ ANSWERS AND EXPLANATIONS

1. **C** The periodontal ligament is derived from the dental sac, a capsule-like structure that develops from the mesenchyme surrounding the tooth.

2. **B** The odontoblasts derived from mesenchymal cells in the dental papilla (future pulp) give rise to predentin and deposit it adjacent to the inner enamel epithelium. Later, the predentin calcifies and becomes dentin.

3. **D** Cells of the inner enamel epithelium adjacent to the dentin differentiate into ameloblasts. These cells produce enamel in the form of prisms (rods) and deposit it over the dentin.

4. **A** The dental pulp derived from the mesenchymal dental papilla of the embryo contains the vessels and nerves of the tooth.

5. **D** The ameloblasts are enamel formers. They produce long enamel prisms and deposit them over the dentin. Enamel formation begins at about 20 weeks in the deciduous teeth and continues in the permanent teeth until about age 16. If vitamin D is deficient during this period, the erupted surfaces of the teeth may be rough instead of smooth and shiny. The ameloblastic layer also induces the odontoblastic layer to form. Hence, if the ameloblasts do not differentiate normally (e.g.,

as in vitamin A deficiency), dentin formation is also affected.

6. **E** The inner cells of the dental sac differentiate into cementoblasts, which produce cementum and deposit it over the dentin of the root.

7. **C** The inner enamel epithelium of the enamel organ induces the adjacent mesenchymal cells in the dental papilla to differentiate into an odontoblastic layer. The inner enamel epithelium differentiates into ameloblasts, the enamel-forming cells.

8. **E** The dental sac develops from the mesenchyme that surrounds the developing tooth. This capsule-like structure gives rise to cementoblasts, which form cementum, and to the periodontal ligament, which embeds in the cementum and the surrounding bony socket of the tooth. Thus, the periodontal ligament holds the tooth in its socket.

9. **A** The dental lamina develops from the oral ectoderm and gives rise to the deciduous and permanent tooth buds.

10. **D** The dental papilla, a condensation of mesenchyme, invaginates the tooth bud, giving it the appearance of a cap. The dental papilla gives rise to the dental pulp and to the odontoblasts, which

Answers and Explanations *Continued*

form the dentin. There is some evidence that the mesenchymal cells that differentiate into odontoblasts are derived from the neural crest.

11. **B** The tooth buds for the permanent teeth develop from continuations of the dental laminae. They begin to appear at about 10 weeks and lie lingual to the deciduous tooth buds.

12. **C** The inner enamel epithelium is part of the enamel organ. Other parts are the outer enamel epithelium and the enamel reticulum. For a while, the enamel organ is attached to the oral epithelium by the dental lamina.

13. **D** Melanocytes differentiate from melanoblasts, which are derived from neural crest cells. Melanoblasts migrate into the dermis during the early fetal period and soon enter the epidermis where they slowly differentiate into melanocytes. These cells produce melanin and distribute it to the epidermal cells after birth. Melanoblasts also migrate into the hair bulbs and differentiate into melanocytes. Melanin is distributed to the hair-forming cells before birth.

14. **B** The ameloblastic layer induces the mesenchymal cells in the dental papilla adjacent to the inner enamel epithelium to differentiate into odontoblasts. If there is a deficiency of vitamin A, the ameloblasts do not differentiate properly. Consequently, there is abnormal formation of odontoblasts.

15. **C** Lanugo is the soft downy hairs that are first produced by the hair follicles. These hairs are chiefly shed before or right after birth and are replaced by coarser hairs that arise from new hair follicles.

16. **A** Tetracycline antibiotics are known to cause brownish yellow discoloration and fetal enamel hypoplasia if given to pregnant females or to children. If given after the eighth year, the third molar teeth are the only ones that may be affected because they are still developing.

17. **C** Most sebaceous glands arise as buds from the sides of the epithelial root sheaths of hair follicles, late in the second trimester of pregnancy. A few sebaceous glands develop from the epidermis, independently of hair follicles (e.g., in the eyelids and labia minora).

18. **E** The inner and outer enamel epithelia of the enamel organ come together and fuse in the neck region of the tooth, where they form the epithelial root sheath. This sheath grows into the mesenchyme and initiates root formation.

19. **B** The ameloblastic layer is derived from the inner enamel epithelium of the enamel organ. The ameloblasts produce enamel and deposit it over the dentin. As the enamel increases, the ameloblasts regress toward the outer enamel epithelium. Enamel and dentin formation begins at the tip (cusp) of the tooth and progresses toward the future root.

20. **D** Neural crest cells are derived from the neuroepithelium of the neural plate. When the neural folds fuse, some neuroectodermal cells at the lateral edges of the neural plate are not incorporated into the neural tube; these cells form the neural crest that gives rise to neural crest cells.

■ NOTES

Review Examination

The following multiple-choice questions are based on all chapters in this study guide and review manual. You should be able to answer these questions in one and a half hours. The key to the correct responses is on page 196.

■ FIVE-CHOICE COMPLETION QUESTIONS

Directions: Each of the following statements or questions is followed by five suggested responses or completions. **Select the one best answer** in each case.

1. Which statement about a 14-day blastocyst is *false*?
   A. Extraembryonic coelom surrounds the yolk sac.
   B. Chorionic villi are absent.
   C. A primordial uteroplacental circulation is established.
   D. The extraembryonic mesoderm is split into two layers.
   E. None of the above.

2. Morphologically abnormal sperms are believed to cause
   A. monosomy
   B. congenital abnormalities
   C. trisomy
   D. Klinefelter syndrome
   E. none of the above

3. The notochordal process lengthens by addition of cells from the
   A. notochord
   B. primitive streak
   C. notochordal plate
   D. primitive node
   E. primitive groove

4. During the early part of the fourth week, the rate of growth at the periphery of the embryonic disc fails to keep pace with rate of growth of the
   A. yolk sac
   B. neural tube
   C. embryonic coelom
   D. amniotic cavity
   E. primitive gut

5. Derivatives of the first pharyngeal pouch include
   A. tympanic antrum
   B. tubotympanic recess
   C. tympanic cavity
   D. pharyngotympanic tube
   E. all the above

Five-Choice Completion Questions *Continued*

6. Known causes of microcephaly include each of the following *except*
   - A. rubella (German measles)
   - B. cytomegalovirus
   - C. thalidomide
   - D. therapeutic radiation
   - E. *Toxoplasma gondii*

7. Each of the following would be good advice to give a woman who has just missed a menstrual period and may be pregnant *except*
   - A. obtain a vaccination against rubella infection.
   - B. avoid exposure to radiation whether for diagnostic or therapeutic purposes.
   - C. do not take any drugs that are not prescribed by a medical doctor.
   - D. stay away from people with infectious diseases.
   - E. eat a good-quality diet and do not smoke.

8. An examination of the placenta and fetal membranes of male twins revealed two amnions, two chorions, and fused placentas. Twinning probably resulted from
   - A. dispermy
   - B. fertilization of two ova
   - C. superfecundation
   - D. fertilization of one ovum
   - E. treatment with gonadotropins

9. Structures derived from the fourth pair of pharyngeal pouches include
   - A. Hassall corpuscles
   - B. thymus gland
   - C. superior parathyroid glands
   - D. inferior parathyroid glands
   - E. all the above

10. The right auricle of the heart is derived from the
    - A. primitive pulmonary vein
    - B. sinus venosus
    - C. right pulmonary vein
    - D. sinus venarum
    - E. primordial atrium

11. Each of the following structures is part of the first pharyngeal arch *except* the
    - A. facial nerve
    - B. mandibular prominence
    - C. Meckel cartilage
    - D. primordium of the malleus
    - E. maxillary prominence

12. In humans, cleft lip, with or without cleft palate, usually results from
    - A. riboflavin deficiency
    - B. infectious diseases
    - C. irradiation
    - D. cortisone
    - E. mutant genes

13. Which of the following is most likely to cause severe congenital anomalies in human embryos?
    - A. Cortisone
    - B. Potassium iodide
    - C. Aminopterin
    - D. Lysergic acid
    - E. Norethynodrel

Five-Choice Completion Questions *Continued*

14. The most distinctive characteristic of a primary chorionic villus is its
    A. outer syncytial layer
    B. cytotrophoblastic core
    C. villous appearance
    D. mesenchymal core
    E. cytotrophoblastic shell

15. A neonate with ambiguous genitalia was found to have chromatin-negative nuclei. Gonads were palpable in the inguinal canals. The phallus was short and curved (chordee). There was no family history of intersexuality. What is the most likely diagnosis?
    A. Perineal hypospadias
    B. Gonadal dysgenesis
    C. Male pseudohermaphroditism
    D. Female pseudohermaphroditism
    E. True hermaphroditism

16. Amniocentesis and amniotic fluid examination are most commonly used to
    A. diagnose chromosomal sex
    B. detect placental insufficiency
    C. determine the composition of the fluid
    D. detect chromosomal abnormalities
    E. diagnose a multiple gestation

17. Narrowing of the lumen in pyloric stenosis usually results from
    A. hypertrophy of the longitudinal muscular layer
    B. a diaphragm-like narrowing of the pyloric lumen
    C. persistence of the solid stage of pyloric development
    D. hypertrophy of the circular muscular layer
    E. fetal vascular accident

18. Which of the following cells produce pulmonary surfactant?
    A. Type I alveolar epithelial cells
    B. Type II alveolar epithelial cells
    C. Alveolar macrophages (phagocytes)
    D. Pulmonary epithelial cells
    E. Endothelial cells

19. You examine a neonate and observe ambiguous external genitalia. Buccal smears show chromatin-positive nuclei. Then you detect an elevated 17-ketosteroid output. What is the most likely diagnosis?
    A. Gonadal dysgenesis resulting from chromosomal abnormalities
    B. Female pseudohermaphroditism caused by maternal androgens
    C. Congenital virilizing adrenocortical hyperplasia
    D. Male infant with perineal hypospadias
    E. Familial male pseudohermaphroditism

20. Anorectal agenesis usually is associated with a rectourethral fistula. The embryologic basis of the fistula is
    A. abnormal partitioning of the cloaca
    B. agenesis of the urorectal septum
    C. failure of fixation of the hindgut
    D. failure of the proctodeum to develop
    E. premature rupture of the anal membrane

Five-Choice Completion Questions *Continued*

21. Congenital heart disease most frequently results from
    A. maternal medications
    B. rubella virus
    C. mutant genes
    D. fetal distress
    E. genetic and environmental factors

22. The primordial germ cells are first observed in the
    A. dorsal mesentery
    B. primary sex cords
    C. gonadal ridges
    D. wall of the yolk sac
    E. mesoderm of the allantois

23. As the metanephric diverticulum grows it becomes capped by _____ mesoderm.
    A. splanchnic
    B. mesonephric
    C. metanephric
    D. somatic
    E. intermediate

24. The most common type of anorectal anomaly is
    A. anal stenosis
    B. anorectal agenesis
    C. ectopic anus
    D. anal agenesis
    E. persistent anal membrane

25. The most common cause of female pseudohermaphroditism is
    A. androgenic hormone ingestion
    B. adrenocortical hyperplasia
    C. arrhenoblastoma in the mother
    D. testicular feminization
    E. maternal progestins

26. A fetus born prematurely during which of the following periods of lung development may survive?
    A. Organogenetic
    B. Canalicular
    C. Pseudoglandular
    D. Terminal sac
    E. Embryonic

27. Exstrophy of the bladder often is associated with
    A. adrenocortical hyperplasia
    B. epispadias
    C. hypospadias
    D. urachal fistula
    E. chromosomal abnormalities

28. The most common congenital anomaly of the heart and great vessels associated with the congenital rubella syndrome is
    A. coarctation of the aorta
    B. tetralogy of Fallot
    C. patent ductus arteriosus
    D. atrial septal defect
    E. ventricular septal defect

29. The mesonephric duct in male embryos gives rise to the
    A. ductus deferens
    B. duct of Gartner
    C. ductuli efferentes
    D. duct of epoophoron
    E. rete testis

ANGLO-EUROPEAN COLLEGE OF CHIROPRACTIC

Five-Choice Completion Questions *Continued*

30. Hematopoiesis begins during the _____ week of development.
    - A. third
    - B. fourth
    - C. fifth
    - D. sixth
    - E. seventh

31. The most common type of accessory rib is
    - A. cervical
    - B. sacral
    - C. fused
    - D. thoracic
    - E. lumbar

32. The ameloblasts of the developing tooth produce
    - A. predentin
    - B. dentin
    - C. cementum
    - D. enamel
    - E. periodontium

33. Which of the following structures is *not* derived from mesoderm?
    - A. Choroid
    - B. Membranous labyrinth
    - C. Extrinsic eye muscles
    - D. Sclera
    - E. Bony labyrinth

34. The myelin sheath of a peripheral nerve fiber is formed by
    - A. mesenchymal cells
    - B. neuroepithelial cells
    - C. Schwann cells
    - D. neural crest cells
    - E. microglia

35. Teratogens acting after the _____ week do not cause severe limb defects.
    - A. second
    - B. third
    - C. fourth
    - D. fifth
    - E. sixth

36. At birth, the inferior end of the spinal cord usually lies at the level of the _____ vertebra.
    - A. first sacral
    - B. third sacral
    - C. first lumbar
    - D. third lumbar
    - E. twelfth thoracic

37. Structures derived from ectoderm include
    - A. external acoustic meatus
    - B. otic vesicle
    - C. corneal epithelium
    - D. lens
    - E. all the above

38. Cellular components of the retina derived from the internal layer of the optic cup include
    - A. rod cells
    - B. ganglion cells
    - C. neuroglial cells
    - D. bipolar cells
    - E. all the above

Five-Choice Completion Questions *Continued*

39. The myelin sheaths surrounding axons in the central nervous system are formed by
    A. neuroglial cells
    B. astrocytes
    C. oligodendrocytes
    D. microglial cells
    E. Schwann cells

40. Myoblasts from the occipital myotomes give rise to muscles of the
    A. neck
    B. ear
    C. eye
    D. tongue
    E. pharynx

41. Most congenital anomalies of teeth are caused by
    A. rubella virus
    B. genetic factors
    C. tetracyclines
    D. irradiation
    E. syphilis

42. Conditions known to follow infection with cytomegalovirus or *Toxoplasma gondii* during the fetal period include
    A. mental retardation
    B. hydrocephaly
    C. microcephaly
    D. microphthalmia
    E. all the above

■ FIVE-CHOICE ASSOCIATION QUESTIONS

Directions: Each group of questions below consists of a numbered list of descriptive words or phrases accompanied by a diagram with certain parts indicated by letters or by a list of lettered headings. For each numbered word or phrase, **select the lettered part or heading** that matches it correctly and then insert the letter in the space to the right of the appropriate number. Sometimes more than one numbered word or phrase may be correctly matched to the same lettered part or heading.

A. Allantois
B. Primitive streak
C. Notochord
D. Blood island
E. Neural plate

43. _____ Gives rise to the brain and spinal cord
44. _____ Source of mesenchyme
45. _____ Rudimentary structure
46. _____ Appears in the wall of the yolk sac

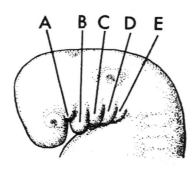

47. _____ Its muscle element gives rise to the muscles of facial expression
48. _____ Its cartilage forms a greater cornu of the hyoid bone
49. _____ Its cartilage gives rise to the styloid process
50. _____ Forms the inferior part of the face
51. _____ Gives rise to the lateral palatine process
52. _____ Supplied by the vagus nerve

Five-Choice Association Questions *Continued*

A. Valve of the foramen ovale
B. Partitions primitive atrium
C. Crista dividens
D. Foramen ovale
E. Umbilical vein

53. _____ Its inferior edge directs blood to the left atrium
54. _____ Carries well-oxygenated blood to the fetus
55. _____ Remains of the septum primum
56. _____ Opening in the septum secundum
57. _____ Early septum primum
58. _____ Part of the septum secundum

59. _____ Its free border contains the umbilical vein
60. _____ Embryonic site of hematopoiesis
61. _____ Derived from the foregut and midgut
62. _____ Hepatoduodenal ligament

A. Scaphocephaly
B. Apical ectodermal ridge
C. Somite
D. Meromelia
E. Hemivertebra

63. _____ Exerts an inductive influence during limb development
64. _____ Craniosynostosis
65. _____ Partial absence of a limb
66. _____ Limb muscles
67. _____ Scoliosis
68. _____ Premature closure of sagittal suture

69. _____ Gives rise to the lens
70. _____ Future optic nerve
71. _____ Differentiates into nonpigmented portion of the ciliary epithelium
72. _____ Becomes pigmented layer of the retina
73. _____ Optic fissure
74. _____ Becomes specialized for sensitivity to light

A. Neural crest
B. Alar plates
C. Basal plates
D. Neuroepithelium
E. Spinal ganglion cells

75. _____ Gracile nuclei
76. _____ Form ventral gray columns
77. _____ Neuroglia
78. _____ Unipolar afferent neurons

■ KEY TO CORRECT RESPONSES

1. B	14. B	27. B	40. D	53. C	66. C
2. E	15. A	28. C	41. B	54. E	67. E
3. D	16. D	29. A	42. E	55. A	68. A
4. B	17. D	30. A	43. E	56. D	69. D
5. E	18. B	31. E	44. B	57. B	70. A
6. C	19. C	32. D	45. A	58. C	71. C
7. A	20. A	33. B	46. D	59. E	72. B
8. B	21. E	34. C	47. C	60. D	73. E
9. C	22. D	35. C	48. D	61. B	74. C
10. E	23. C	36. D	49. C	62. A	75. B
11. A	24. B	37. E	50. B	63. B	76. C
12. E	25. B	38. E	51. A	64. A	77. D
13. C	26. D	39. C	52. E	65. D	78. E

■ INTERPRETATION OF YOUR SCORE

Number of Correct Responses	*Level of Performance*
70–78	Excellent–Exceptional
55–69	Superior–Very Superior
43–54	Average–Above Average
37–42	Poor–Marginal
36 or less	Very Poor–Failure

ANGLO-EUROPEAN COLLEGE OF CHIROPRACTIC